AF526854

Practical Physiology

RECORD BOOK

Student's Name: ____________________

Roll No. ____________________ **Year/Session:** ____________________

University Roll No. ____________________

College ____________________

This is to certify that this is a bonafide record of work done by ____________________ during the year 20....–20..... His/her work is complete/incomplete/satisfactory/fair/good.

____
Signature of Staff in charge

____
Signature of Prof. & HOD

Submitted for University Examination in Practical Physiology 20________

Examiners: ____________________ ____________________

LABORATORY DISCIPLINE

Planning, experimentation and observation are central concepts to all scientific advancement. Students are therefore required to

- Read up relevant material on the practical for proper conduct of the experiment.
- Collect the equipment needed for the experiment from the laboratory staff, which should be returned in good condition at the end of the practical.
- Wear a clean white laboratory coat and have the following instruments: knee hammer, pen torch and measuring tape, stethoscope.
- Keep the work area neat and clean during the practical
- If in doubt, consult the instructor, without disturbing other students in the laboratory.

REPORT OF DATA AND PRACTICAL EVALUATION

- Results or data collected by practical work should be neatly entered in observation notebook. The data should be presented to the concerned instructor and their signature taken before leaving the laboratory.
- Answer the questions given at the end of each experiment in the record. These are intended to stimulate further study, thereby assisting the learning process.
- Evaluation of the practical work for internal assessment will be based on periodic practical evaluation (20 marks) and the laboratory record (5 marks)
- During the session, 4–6 practical examinations will be conducted for the purpose of evaluation. Practical examinations for internal assessment will be in the form of Major Experiment, Minor Experiment, Comments and Calculations.
- The marks for the practical record will be awarded on the basis of neatness, accuracy of work, conduct in the laboratory, the promptness in answering the questions and weekly submission of the record which will be assessed by the instructor.

OUR GOALS

- To provide the student with proper guidance to acquire a hands on knowledge of various laws and physiological principles-through the performance of experiments in physiology.
- To acquire clinical, technical and communication skills and to develop the art of careful observation and precise measurement.
- To acquire training in scientific methods of thought and analysis of data.
- To perform the various experiments, with a high degree of proficiency, in accordance with guidelines laid out by the Medical Council of India for the training of medical professionals.

Other CBS title by the same author

- Review and Physiology

Practical Physiology

RECORD BOOK

M. Chandrasekar MD DA PhD

Professor and Head
Department of Physiology
and
Vice Principal
Meenakshi Medical College and Research Institute
Enathur, Kancheepuram
Tamil Nadu

CBS

CBS Publishers & Distributors Pvt. Ltd.

New Delhi • Bengaluru • Chennai • Kochi • Kolkata • Mumbai
Hyderabad • Nagpur • Patna • Pune • Vijayawada

ISBN: 978-81-239-1950-8

First Edition: 2011
Reprint: 2012, 2014, 2016, 2018, 2019

Published by:
Satish Kumar Jain for CBS Publishers & Distributors Pvt. Ltd.,
4819/XI Prahlad Street, 24 Ansari Road, Daryaganj, New Delhi - 110002
delhi@cbspd.com, cbspubs@airtelmail.in • www.cbspd.com
Ph.: 23289259, 23266861, 23266867 • Fax: 011-23243014

Corporate Office: 204 FIE, Industrial Area, Patparganj, Delhi - 110 092
Ph: 49344934 • E-mail: publishing@cbspd.com • publicity@cbspd.com

Branches:
- ***Bengaluru:*** 2975, 17th Cross, K.R. Road, Bansankari 2nd Stage, Bengaluru - 70 • Ph: +91-80-26771678/79 • Fax: +91-80-26771680 E-mail: cbsbng@gmail.com, bangalore@cbspd.com
- ***Chennai:*** No. 7, Subbaraya Street, Shenoy Nagar, Chennai - 600030 Ph: +91-44-26681266, 26680620 • E-mail: chennai@cbspd.com
- ***Kochi:*** Ashana House, 39/1904, A.M. Thomas Road, Valanjambalam, Ernakulum, Kochi • Ph: +91-484-4059061-65 Fax: +91-484-4059065 • E-mail: cochin@cbspd.com
- ***Kolkata:*** 6-B, Ground Floor, Rameshwar Shaw Road, Kolkata - 700014 Ph: +91-33-22891126/7/8 • E-mail: kolkata@cbspd.com
- ***Mumbai:*** 83-C, Dr. E. Moses Road, Worli, Mumbai - 400018 Ph: +91-9833017933, 022-24902340/41 • E-mail: mumbai@cbspd.com

Representatives:
- Hyderabad: 0-9885175004
- Nagpur: 0-9021734563
- Patna: 0-9334159340
- Pune: 0-9623451994
- Vijayawada: 0-9000660880

Printed at: India Binding House, Noida, UP (India)

Preface

To know clinical medicine and its applications, understanding of human physiology is a must. As the medical education is shifting from discipline-based learning to problem-based learning, simultaneous learning and training on various systems and diseases of the body become mandatory.

The extent and magnitude of developments in physiology and medicine necessitate the revision or upgradation of any scientific knowledge within a few years. The success of the first edition of this practical physiology record book evidenced by several reprints in a few years has prompted me to work for the second edition. I have received several meaningful suggestions from our peers, colleagues, and students, which form the basis of this revision.

I hope that this fully revised edition will meet the expectations of the physiology faculty and students and they will continue to give their valuable inputs in improving the practical book further in subsequent printings and editions.

M. Chandrasekar MD DA PhD
Professor and Head
Department of Physiology
and Vice Principal
Meenakshi Medical College and Research Institute
Enathur, Kanchipuram, Talim Nadu

Contents

Preface ... *v*

HAEMATOLOGY EXPERIMENTS

1. The Compound Microscope ... 1
2. Blood Sample Collection ... 7
3. The Haemocytometer ... 9
4. Enumeration of RBC ... 13
5. Estimation of Haemoglobin ... 19
6. Packed Cell Volume and Calculation of Blood Indices ... 23
7. Determination of ESR ... 27
8. Total Leucocyte Count ... 33
9. Differential Count of White Blood Cells ... 37
10. Absolute Eosinophil Count ... 47
11. Determination of Bleeding Time and Clotting Time ... 51
12. Blood Grouping ... 57
13. Osmotic Fragility of Red Blood Cells ... 61
14. Specific Gravity of Blood ... 65

CLINICAL PHYSIOLOGY

1. General Examination ... 69
2. Examination of the Respiratory System ... 75
3. Recording of Respiratory Movements (Stethography) ... 83
4. Spirometry ... 87
5. Respiratory Efficiency Tests ... 91
6. Examination of the Cardiovascular System ... 93
7. Determination of the Blood Pressure ... 101
8. Electrocardiography ... 107
9. Examination of Sensory System ... 111
10. Examination of Motor System ... 117
11. Reflexes ... 129
12. Examination of Cranial Nerves I to VI ... 137
13. Examination of Cranial Nerves VII to XII ... 149
14. Perimetry ... 159
15. Cerebellar Function Tests ... 161

Comments ... 165

Calculations ... 194

Haematology Experiments

Experiment 1: The Compound Microscope

Aim of the Experiment

To study the parts of a compound microscope and to view slides under the microscope.

Apparatus Required

Compound microscope, cedar wood oil, stained slides, blood film and light source.

Parts of the Compound Microscope

A typical compound microscope (Fig. 1.1) (synonyms: light microscope, student microscope) consists of the following parts:

1. *The base:* It is 'U' shaped. It serves to support the microscope and provides it with maximum stability.
2. *The pillars:* They are two in number and project upwards from the base and extend up to the handle of the microscope.
3. *The handle:* It is curved and is used to tilt the microscope. It supports the magnifying and adjusting systems.
4. *The body tube or barrel:* It is attached to the handle. It can be raised or lowered while viewing slides. The length of the tube is usually 160 mm.
5. *The adjustment screws:* They include the coarse adjustment screw and the fine adjustment screw. When viewing a slide, the field is initially focussed using the coarse adjustment screw and then fine adjustment should be done.
6. *The stages:* They include the fixed stage and the mechanical stage. The fixed stage is a square platform with an aperture in its centre that allows the light to pass from the light source to the lens The slide to be viewed is placed on this stage. The mechanical stage is fitted on the fixed stage. It is a calibrated metal frame with a spring mounted clip that holds the slide in position. It is fitted with two screws that can be adjusted to move the slide vertically or horizontally.
7. *The nosepiece:* It lies at the lower end of the body tube. It includes:
   a. A fixed nosepiece that is stationary and fitted to the lower end of the body tube.
   b. A revolving nosepiece that lies under the fixed nosepiece. The revolving nosepiece carries the objective lenses. Any lens can be rotated into position as desired. The correct position is indicated by a click.
8. *The objective lenses:* They are three in number and are fitted into the revolving nosepiece. They include:
   a. The low power objective lens, which magnifies the image ten times.
   b. The high power objective lens, which magnifies the image 40 or 45 times.
   c. The oil immersion objective lens that magnifies the image hundred times.

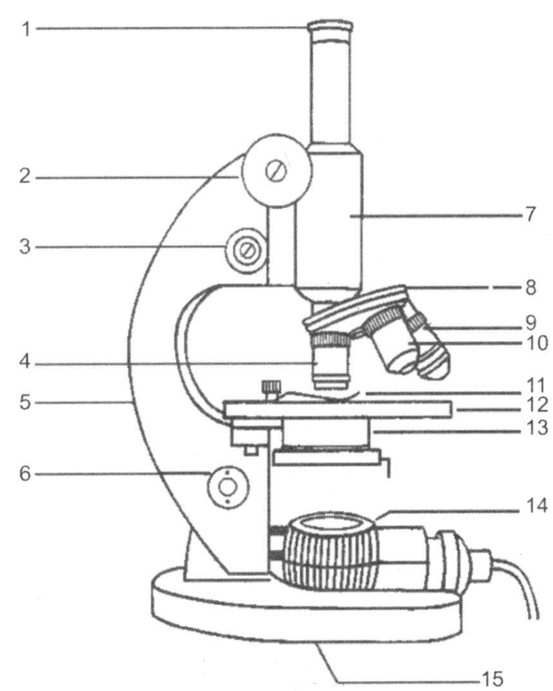

Fig. 1.1: Compound microscope

Student's Notes

9. ***The eyepiece:*** It is fitted into the top of the body tube. Commonly used eyepiece have a magnifying power of ten times.
10. ***The mirror and illumination:*** It lies at the lower end of the microscope just below the condenser. It can be adjusted to reflect light rays into the condenser. The mirror has two surfaces namely a plane surface and a concave surface. The plane mirror is used when the light source is a distant one (e.g. natural day light). The concave mirror is used when the light source is near the microscope (e.g. an electrical lamp). Plane mirror is preferred when viewing an object via oil immersion lens. Certain microscopes have built in electrical light source.
11. ***The condenser:*** It is fitted under the fixed stage and can be raised or lowered using a screw. It has two lenses and an iris diaphragm that can be manipulated to control and amount of light entering the microscope. The condenser functions to convert parallel rays of light reflected from the mirror into a cone or condensed beam of light which then passes towards the stage.
12. ***Working distance:*** It is the distance between objective and slide. It decreases with increasing magnification. For oil immersion 0.15–1.5 mm, High power 0.5–4 mm, Low power 5–15 mm.
13. ***Numerical aperture:*** It is ratio of the diameter of lense to its focal length.

Total Magnification of the Compound Microscope

With an eyepiece of l0X, the magnification provided by a low power objective is 100 times, by a high power objective is 400 times and by oil immersion objective is 1000 times. The maximum effective magnification obtained by compound microscope by altering either the eyepiece or the objective is 1500 times.

The first objective, to be used while viewing a slide, is the low power objective. The microscope is placed in upright position and an appropriate mirror is selected based on the light source. The condenser is lowered and the diaphragm is partly shut to cut down the glare. The slide to be viewed is placed on the fixed stage. The objective is brought to about 1 cm above the slide. Now while looking into the eyepiece, the objective is raised with the coarse adjustment screw till the slide comes into focus. Using the fine adjustment screw, finer details in the slide are focussed.

Having focussed the slide under the low power objective, a greater magnification can be obtained using the high power objective. While using this objective, the condenser is raised and the diaphragm is opened for optimal illumination. The high power objective is swung into position and the area of the slide to be viewed is focussed in a similar manner.

Further magnification can be obtained using the oil immersion objective. A drop of cedar wood oil is placed on the slide and the oil immersion objective is swung into position. The objective is lowered until it touches the oil drop using the coarse adjustment screw. Now the fine adjustment screw is used to obtain a clear image. After use, the lens is cleaned with xylol.

Precautions while using the Compound Microscope

1. While transporting the microscope, one hand is placed under the base and the other hand on the handle. The microscope must not be used by placing it on the edge of the working table.
2. The microscope must not be tilted when counting cells in a counting chamber or when using the oil immersion objectives.
3. The objective must not be moved down while looking into the eyepiece. Such a manoeuvre might risk breaking the slide.
4. All traces of cedar wood oil must be removed from the objective with a clean flannel dipped in xylol.
5. Foreign bodies such as dust must be kept away from the eyepiece and objective.
6. While changing the objective, it should be noted that the objective clicks into its proper position.
7. Examination of the specimen under low and high power should always precede the examination under oil immersion objective.

Other Types of Microscope

1. The simple microscope which refers to a magnifying glass.
2. The binocular microscope which has two eyepieces.
3. The dissection microscope which is a type of binocular used for microdissection.
4. The ultra-microscope which uses ultraviolet light instead of ordinary light and has a magnification of 4000 times.
5. The phase contrast microscope that uses principles of light refraction to produce an image with a good contrast.
6. The fluorescence microscope that uses a fluorescent dye to stain tissues which are studied under the microscope.
7. The transmission electron microscope that uses a beam of electrons instead of light and electron

Student's Notes

magnetic fields instead of glass lenses. This microscope obtains a magnification of up to 1 lakh times.

8. The scanning electron microscope is similar to the transmission electron microscope. It is used for three-dimensional study of surface topography of cells and objects.
9. Dark field microscope—used to study spirochetes in the exudates from leptospiral or syphilitic infection.
10. Interference contrast microscope—useful for wet preparation such as urinary sedements, shower finer details without need of special staining.

QUESTIONS

1. Label the parts of the light/compound microscope in the given diagram.
2. What are the types of microscope?
3. What will be the total magnification—if a low power objective, high power objective or an oil immersion objective is used? (Eyepiece 10 X)
4. What is the function of the condenser?
5. What is the function of the diaphragm?
6. When is concave and plane mirror used?
7. Why should the oil be removed from the oil immersion objective immediately after use?
8. What microscopic adjustments are made when the field of view is not clear?

Student's Notes

Experiment 2: Blood Sample Collection

Aim of the Experiment

To study the different methods of blood collection.

Apparatus Required

Sterile lancet, disposable syringe and needle, anti-coagulant container, cotton spirit.

Procedure

Collections of capillary blood by finger prick method:

1. Clean the tip of the ring or middle finger with a cotton swab dipped in spirit.
2. Allow the finger tip to dry as spirit can cause the haemolysis of blood and pain.
3. Using a sterile lancet prick the finger deep enough to ensure a free flow of blood.

Wipe away the first few drops and collect the sample when the blood is flowing spontaneously. Do not squeeze the finger as tissue fluid can mix with blood and may cause error.

Collection of Venous Blood

Venous blood is usually collected from antecubital vein.

1. Clean the antecubital fossa with spirit and allow it to dry.
2. After applying a tourniquet around the upper arm, introduce a needle under the skin and then puncture the vein from the side. During this procedure, open and close the fist repeatedly so that the vein gets engorged.
3. When the blood flows into the syringe, release the tourniquet and draw the required amount of blood.
4. Withdraw the needle and apply a cotton swab over the site of puncture and apply pressure till the bleeding stops. (To prepare serum, blood can be emptied into a container without anticoagulant. To prepare plasma, blood has to be emptied into a container with anticoagulant.

QUESTIONS

1. What is the difference between serum and plasma?
2. Name the other places for capillary blood withdrawal.
3. Name five commonly used anticoagulants and explain the mode of action.
4. Name any two in vitro and in vivo anticoagulants.
5. Why is the first drop of blood discarded?
6. How does methylated spirit sterilize your finger tip?

Student's Notes

Experiment 3: The Haemocytometer

Aim

To study the working and uses of the haemocytometer.

Principle

A measured unit of blood is diluted quantitatively with diluents by using special measuring devices (pipettes). A mixture of blood and diluting fluid (dilution is known) is released smoothly on to the central platform of the chamber beneath the cover slip (depth of chamber is known). Cells are then counted under this known volume of mixture under the cover slip.

Apparatus Required

Improved Neubauer's counting chamber, RBC pipette, WBC pipette, diluents, cover slip.

Description

The haemocytometer is a box containing all the above apparatus. Improved Neubauer's chamber is a glass slide which has 2 platforms extending across its middle third. These platforms are separated from each other by shallow gutters or trenches. The central platforms are also known as the floor piece. It is 1/10 mm lower than the rest of the slide. The 2 platforms adjacent to the central platform support the slip. When a cover slip is placed in position, a space of 0.1 mm is present between the surface of the floor piece and the under surface of the cover slip.

The central platform has 2 counting grids. Each counting grid has an area 9 mm^2. It is in turn divided into 9 squares with each square having an area of 1 mm^2. The 4 corner squares which are used for WBC counting are each divided by single lines into 16 smaller squares. Each of them has a size measuring 1/4 mm and an area of 1/16 mm^2. The central square which is RBC counting is divided into 25 medium squares each of which is separated from the others by double or triple lines called tram lines. These tram lines extend in all directions. Each of the 25 squares is further divided into 16 small squares by single lines. These are the smallest squares on the grid with each small square having a side measuring 1/20 mm and an area of 1/400 mm^2.

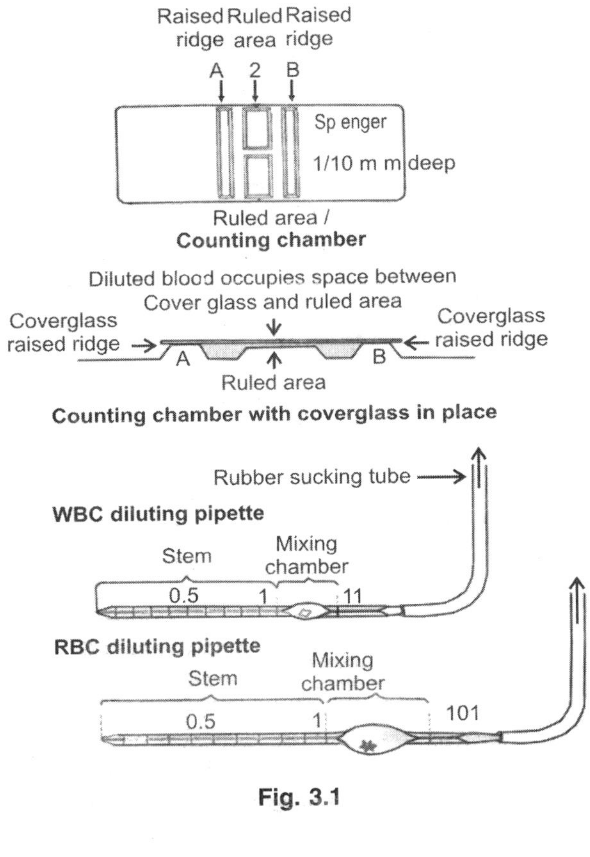

Fig. 3.1

Focussing the Counting Grid

Using the standard protocol, the counting grid is focussed so that the lines are seen clearly. Initially, the lines are focussed under low power. After which, the high power objective is used to view the squares.

Charging the Haemocytometer

A cover slip is placed over the centre of the haemocytometer on top of the pillars. After the blood is well mixed with the diluent, the first two drops are discarded and the pipette is placed on the floor piece so that its tip just touches the edge of the cover slip, at an angle of 30° to the horizontal. The diluted blood is allowed to flow by capillary action evenly and slowly under the cover slip making sure that there is no flow of the mixture into the trenches. If there is over flow of blood into the trenches, the haemocytometer must be charged again after cleaning it. Now the cells are allowed to settle down for 2–3 minutes. After that, the chamber is placed on the microscope. The lines are focussed as desired, depending on the type of cell count after which the chamber is cleaned in running water and dried for reuse.

Student's Notes

THE DILUTING PIPETTES

Introduction

Blood must be adequately diluted before estimating its cell count. This is done using glass capillary pipettes. Knowing the dilution employed, the number of cells in undiluted blood can be calculated.

Description of the Pipettes

There are 2 types of diluting pipettes namely the RBC pipette and the WBC pipette. Each pipette has a long narrow stem with a fine capillary bore and a ground conical tip.

The stem is graduated into 10 parts but has only 2 numbers etched on it namely 0.5 and 1.0 smaller calibrations in tenths allow greater dilutions, if needed. The stem widens into a small bulb which contains a free rolling glass bead, red in RBC pipette and white in WBC pipette. It helps in mixing the blood with the diluting fluid and for quick identification of the pipettes. The volume of the bulb is 10 times the volume of the stem in the WBC pipette, and 100 times the volume of the stem in the RBC pipette. The bulb narrows proximally into a glass capillary to which a long narrow soft rubber tube bearing a mouthpiece is attached. Beyond the bulb, the figure 101 is etched on the RBC pipette and 11 on the WBC pipette.

Filling the Pipette

1. Under aseptic precautions, the finger is pricked and the first 2–3 drops are wiped away following which a good sized drop of free flowing blood is made to form.
2. Holding the mouthpiece between the lips and keeping the pipette horizontal its tip is placed within the edge of the blood drop.
3. Blood is drawn into the pipette by gently sucking on the mouthpiece up to the 0.5 or 1.0 mark depending on the dilution required.
4. The other end of the pipette is tightly closed by clenching the rubber tube.
5. The outside of the pipette tip is wiped (be careful not to touch the tip itself) with cotton and immersed in the diluting fluid while holding.
6. The diluting fluid is sucked up to the 11 mark in case of the WBC pipette or 101 mark in case of the RBC pipette.
7. Dilution of the blood must be done quickly otherwise blood is likely to clot in the stem.
8. Following dilution, the pipette is kept horizontal so that the fluid does not run out.
9. Now by placing the pipette tip against the palm of the left hand and holding it just above the bulb with the thumb and forefinger of the other hand, it is rotated to and fro for 3–4 minutes to allow the mixing of the blood with the diluting fluid.
10. Following this, the counting chamber is charged by discarding the stem fluid (about two drops) and placing the pipette at the edge of the cover slip that lies over counting chamber.

Precautions

1. The pipette must be dry and free from clotted blood and the bead must roll freely.
2. The pipette must be almost horizontal while filling it with blood. The tip must not press against the subject's skin or be lifted out of the blood drop (otherwise air will enter it).
3. The dilution of blood must begin immediately after the blood is drawn or else the blood may clot.
4. Leakage of fluid from the pipette must be avoided while mixing the bulb contents.
5. After charging the haemocytometer, the pipette must be washed in running water following which alcohol is used to remove water. Finally the pipette is washed with acetone to remove the alcohol and left to dry.

QUESTIONS

1. What are the uses of haemocytometer in haematology?
2. How do you identify the RBC and WBC pipette?
3. What are the steps for diluting the blood for various cell counts?
4. What are the precautions taken for pipetting?
5. Why the fluid is not sucked directly from the stock bottle?

Student's Notes

Experiment 4: Enumeration of RBC

Aim

To enumerate the number of red blood cells per cubic millimetre of blood.

Apparatus Required

Haemocytometer, microscope, cover slips, Hayem's fluid, cotton, spirit and lancet.

Composition of Hayem's Fluid

Sodium chloride	: 0.5 g to maintain isotonicity
Sodium sulphate	: 2.5 g to prevent rouleaux formation
Mercuric chloride	: 0.25 g to fix the cells and act as a preservative.
Distilled water	: 100 ml

Principle

The number of red cells in the blood is too many and the size of the cells is too small. It is therefore not possible to count the cells even under high power. This difficulty is overcome by diluting the blood to a known degree.

Procedure

Collection and Dilution of Blood

The RBC pipette is cleaned with distilled water, alcohol and finally with ether and dried. Sterilize the tip of the middle finger of left hand. A prick is made in the finger to a depth of 3–4 mm with a sterile lancet. The pricking should be done only in the middle or ring finger. Never use the thumb or index finger because the tendon is superficial. Blood is drawn up to 0.5 unit followed by the diluting fluid up to 101 units without any air bubble. Mixing is done by rotating the pipette between the palms. After mixing the blood with diluting fluid, keep it aside for 3 minutes.

Microscopic Adjustments

1. The cells are focussed under low power and ultimately the counting is done under high power.
2. Concave mirror to be used.
3. Condenser to be lowered.
4. Diaphragm is adjusted for adequate entry of light. Focus the RBC rulings under low power. Place the cover slip over the raised ridges.

Discard the fluid from the stem of the pipette. Keeping it at 30°–45°, charge the fluid from the bulb between the cover slip and the central platform, so that it spreads uniformly. Care is taken not to induce any air bubbles. Wait for 2–3 minutes for the cells to settle down.

Counting the Cells

Cells are to be counted from four corners and one central medium square of the RBC rulings. Each medium square is made up of 16 smaller squares. While counting, the cells lying inside as well as on the upper and left border of the smallest square are to be taken into account. In total the cells lying in the 80 smallest squares has to be counted.

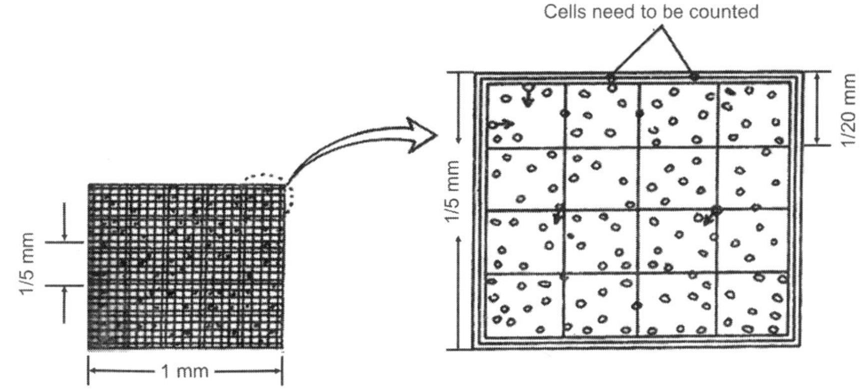

Fig. 4.1

Student's Notes

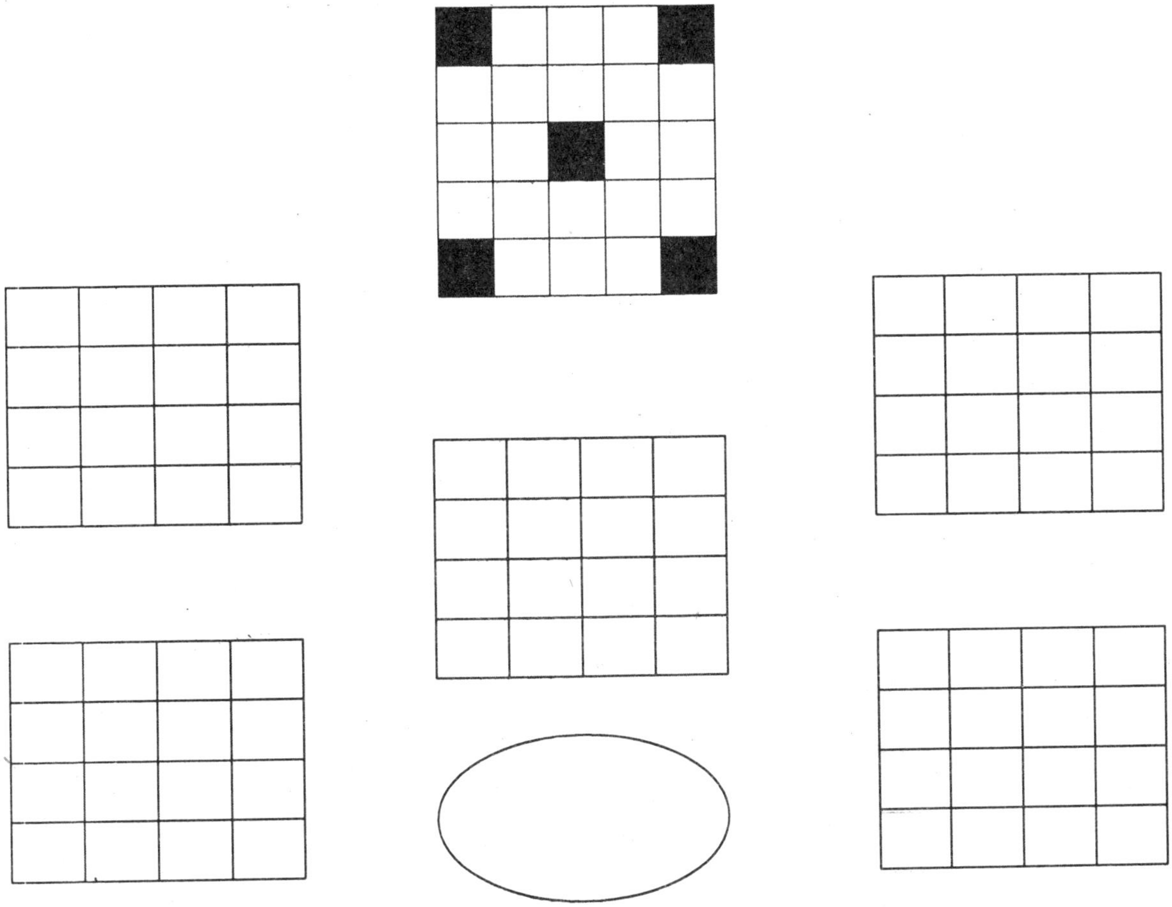

Total no of cells in 80 small squares =
Draw a neat diagram of an RBC in the circle

Fig. 4.2: RBC count

Calculation

Area of 1 medium square	$= 1/25\ mm^2\ (1/5 \times 1/5)$
Depth of the chamber	$= 1/10$ mm
Volume of the fluid over 1 medium square	$= 1/25 \times 1/10$
	$= 1/250\ mm^3$
Volume of fluid present over 5 medium squares	$= 1/250 \times 5$
	$= 1/50\ mm^3$
Number of RBC counted from 5 medium squares, i.e. in $1/50\ mm^3$ of diluted blood	= N
Number of RBC in $1\ mm^3$ of diluted blood	$= N \times 50$
Dilution factor	= 1:200
Number of RBC in $1\ mm^3$ of undiluted blood	$= N \times 50 \times 200$
	$= 10000 \times N$

Precautions

1. Finger should not be squeezed once pricked, because the interstitial fluid will mix with blood and give wrong value.
2. As soon as prick was given, the blood should be immediately diluted with the RBC diluting fluid to prevent clotting.
3. There should not be any air bubbles in the pipette when blood or diluting fluid is sucked.
4. Do not tilt the microscope.
5. Cover slip should be placed uniformly over the ridges.
6. During charging, care should be taken to prevent fluid from entering into the trenches.

Discussion

Normal value

Male	4.5–6.0 million/cu mm
Female	4.0–5.5 million/cu mm

Student's Notes

Physiological Variation

1. *Diurnal variation:* Variation of about 5% may occur per period of 24 hours. The count is least during sleep and maximum during evenings.
2. *Muscular exercise:* The count increases temporarily due to hypoxic stimulus.
3. *Altitudes:* RBC count increases with increase in altitude.
4. *High external temperature:* RBC count increases with increase of temperature. RBC count also depends on the age and sex of a person.

Pathological Variations

Anaemia: It means a significant reduction in number of red cells and/or the amount of haemoglobin in the blood as compared to the normal state.

Polycythemia: An increase in the number of red cells is called polycythemia. It may be due to:

1. Emphysema
2. Congenital heart disease
3. Poisoning by chemicals like arsenic and phosphorus.
4. Repeated small haemorrhages.

A common type of secondary polycythemia occurs in natives who live in high altitudes. The blood count may be 6 to 7 millions/cu mm.

Polycythemia vera: It is a primary condition due to alteration in the haemocytoblastic cell. RBC count may be 7–8 millions/cu mm.

Result

The RBC count of the given subject is ....

QUESTIONS

1. During dilution, blood is drawn up to the 0.5 mark and dilution fluid up to the 101 mark. Yet why do we say the dilution is 1:200? (and not 1:202).
2. While mixing the fluids, why should you never shake the pipette in the direction of its long axis?
3. Why is it important to discard the first few drops from the pipette before charging the counting chamber?
4. What is the normal range of erythrocyte count?
5. What are the physiological variations in RBC count?
6. Explain the terms "anaemia" and "polycythemia" and classify in brief their various types. Describe the terms "physiological anaemia of pregnancy" and "reticulocyte response".
7. What is the most powerful stimulus for RBC production?
8. What is the normal size of RBC. Name one condition when RBC size is less than normal and one condition where the RBC size is more than normal?
9. What will happen, if the RBC pipette is not dry before the experiment?
10. What is polycythemia vera rubra?
11. What is the composition and function of Hayem's fluid?
12. What happens to leucocytes when blood is mixed with diluting fluid?
13. What is the morphology of RBC and why?
14. What is rouleax formation?
15. Mention the lifespan of RBCs.
16. Enumerate the functions of RBCs.

Student's Notes

Experiment 5: Estimation of Haemoglobin

Aim

To estimate the amount of haemoglobin in 100 ml of blood by Sahli's method.

Principle

The haemoglobin present in a measured sample of blood is converted by dilute HCl to acid haematin which is brown in colour. The intensity of this colour depends on the amount of acid haematin which in turn depends on the haemoglobin. The colour of this solution is compared with that of a standard by direct vision.

Apparatus

Sahli's haemoglobinometer (haemometer)—which consists of:

1. *Comparator*—a rectangular plastic box with a slot which accommodates the Hb tube and non-fading standard fixed on either side in front of an opaque white glass.
2. *Haemoglobin tube*—graduated in g% (2–24 g%) on one side and in percentage (20–140%) on the other.
3. *Haemoglobin pipette* with a 20 cu mm mark and rubber tubing with a mouthpiece.
4. A glass rod to stir.
5. N/10 hydrochloric acid.
6. Distilled water.
7. Lancet, cotton and spirit.

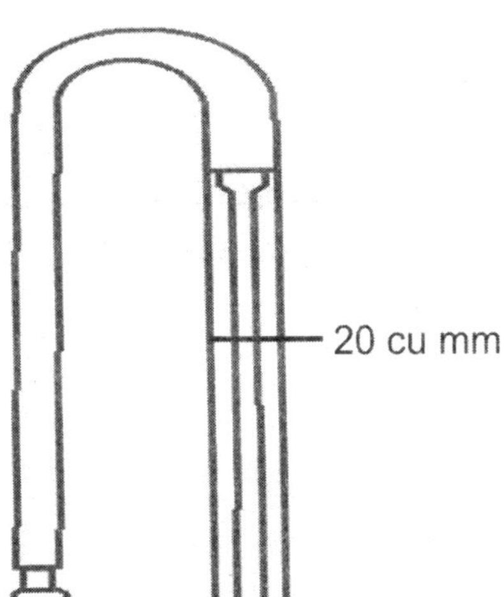

Fig. 5.1: Haemoglobin pipette

Procedure

1. N/10 HCl is taken up to the lowest mark in the graduated tube.
2. The finger is pricked under aseptic precautions.
3. The pipette is filled with blood up to 20 cu mm mark taking care not to allow air bubbles to enter.
4. After wiping the blood sticking to the outside of the pipette, its tip is dipped in the acid and the blood is expelled.
5. The pipette is rinsed 3 or 4 times with the acid solution, till all the blood is washed out.
6. The blood and the acid are mixed well with the glass rod. The tube is allowed to stand for 8–10 min for the formation of acid haematin.
7. Distilled water is added drop by drop, mixed well and the colour is compared with that of the standard.
8. Care should be taken to remove the glass rod while matching and not to view through the graduations.
9. This is continued till the colour matches.
10. The lowest point of the meniscus is read which directly gives the haemoglobin concentration in 100 ml of blood.

Precautions

1. All precautions mentioned for collection of blood and filling the pipette should be observed.
2. Enough time should be allowed for conversion of all the Hb into acid haematin.
3. The solution must be properly mixed.
4. Colour matching should not be delayed and should be done in bright light.

Disadvantages of Sahli's Method

1. As acid haematin is not true solution, some turbidity may result.
2. The method estimates only oxy Hb and reduced Hb.
3. The colour of the glass standards may fade over time.

Advantages of Sahli's Method

1. Easy to perform.
2. Economical.
3. Less time consuming.

Result

The haemoglobin content of the given subject is ...... gm/100 ml.

Student's Notes

QUESTIONS

1. What is the normal range of the haemoglobin in blood?
2. Record the Hb content of your blood. Is it normal?
3. Comment on the results of your group. Are there any abnormal values? Are there any attributable causes for the above mentioned?
4. Name the other methods to estimate haemoglobin?
5. What is the oxygen carrying capacity of the blood?
6. What is the colour in the haemoglobinometer due to .... ?
7. What are the functions of N/10 HCl in this experiment?
8. What are the advantages of doing red cell indices?
9. What is a picogram?
10. What is the structure of haemoglobin? What is it made up of?
11. Discuss the physiological factors which influence the Hb content of blood.
12. Define anaemia.
13. List 4 pathological conditions where the Hb content is altered.

Student's Notes

Experiment 6: Packed Cell Volume and Calculation of Blood Indices

Aim

To find out the packed cell volume. And then ....To calculate the following blood indices.

1. Colour index
2. Mean corpuscular volume
3. Mean corpuscular haemoglobin and
4. Mean corpuscular haemoglobin concentration.

Apparatus Required

Centrifuge machine, haematocrit tube (Wintrobe's), Pasteur's pipette, syringe with needle, EDTA or double oxalate crystals, etc.

Principle

When blood is mixed with an anticoagulant is centrifuged in a haematocrit tube, the corpuscles settle at the bottom and the ratio of packed red cells to that of whole volume in the haematocrit tube is called packed cell volume or haematocrit volume of blood.

Procedure

1. Macro haematocrit method—Wintrobe's method.
2. Micro haematocrit method—Using capillary tube (most accurate method).

Macro haematocrit method—Wintrobe's method (this is followed in lab): In a clean dry syringe 2 ml of blood was drawn from the antecubital vein and mixed with double oxalate. The blood was then filled in the haematocrit tube up to the mark '0' using a Pasteur's pipette. The tube was centrifuged at the rate of 3,000 revolutions per minute for a period of 30 minutes. The packed cell volume was read in percentage directly.

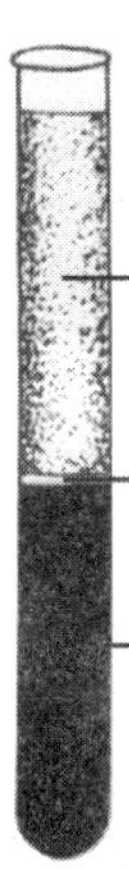

Plasma (52–57%)
Buffy coat (1%)
WBC and platelets
Red cells (43–47%)

Fig. 6.1: Layers of normal blood after centrifugation

Normal values	*Average*	*Range*
Adult men	45%	40–50%
Adult women	42%	37–47%

Result

PCV of the given blood sample is ....

CALCULATION OF BLOOD INDICES

Following values are referred as RBC indices or haematological indices.

1. Mean corpuscular volume (MCV).
2. Mean corpuscular haemoglobin (MCH).
3. Mean corpuscular haemoglobin concentration (MCHC).
4. Colour index.

MCV, MCH and MCHC are referred as absolute values. These values are widely used for the classification of anaemia.

To calculate the blood indices, the RBC count and haemoglobin content are essential. For RBC count and haemoglobin content, the values are taken from the results of 4 and 5, respectively.

This is the value of my blood

PCV =

RBC count =

Haemoglobin content =

1. *Mean corpuscular volume (MCV):* It is the average volume of RBC

$$MCV = \frac{PCV(\text{in percent})}{\text{RBC count in millions / cu mm}} \times 10$$

Normal MCV = 78–96 fL. In microcytic anaemia (iron deficiency) MCV is low. In macrocytic (megaloblastic) anaemia, MCV is increased.

2. *Mean corpuscular haemoglobin (MCH):* Amount of haemoglobin that is present in average RBC.

$$MCH = \frac{Hb(\text{in gm\%})}{\text{RBC count in millions / cu mm}} \times 10$$

Normal range is 27 to 33 picogram. Cells with this value are considered as normochromic.

In iron deficiency anaemia, MCH is low (hypochromic). In megaloblastic anaemia, MCH is high (not hyperchromic why?)

Student's Notes

3. *Mean corpuscular haemoglobin concentration (MCHC):* Average Hb concentration per unit volume of packed RBC.

$$MCHC = \frac{Hb\,(in\,gm\%)}{PCV\,(in\,percent)} \times 100$$

Normal CHC is 30–37 g% (or g /dl). MCHC denotes degree of saturation of Hb in cells. It is the more reliable index than other indices as it dose not involve RBC count for its calculation.

4. *Color index:* Ratio of percentage of Hb to percentage of RBC is called as color index. 14.8 gm% of haemoglobin is considered as 100% and 5 millions/cu mm of RBCs are considered as 100%. Colour index of an individual having haemoglobin 14.8 gm% and RBC 5 million/cu mm will be:

$$MCHC = \frac{Hb\,(in\,gm\%)}{PCV\,(in\%)} \times 100$$

$$= \frac{Hb\,found}{Hb\,normal} \times 100$$

$$= \frac{RBC\,found}{RBC\,normal} \times 100$$

$$Color\,index = \frac{100\%}{100\%} = 1 \text{ or } CI = \frac{Hb\%}{RBC\%}$$

Normal range is 0.85 to 1.1. Color index is useful to know the type of anaemia. Low index indicates hypochromic anaemia.

QUESTIONS

1. How do you do this experiment by micro-haematocrit method?
2. Draw a diagram of the Wintrobe's haematocrit tube showing PCV.
3. Give the significance of PCV.
4. List the physiological conditions where the PCV is increased/decreased.
5. What is the ideal anticoagulant to be used for PCV determination and why?
6. What are the uses of estimation of PCV?
7. Is there any change in PCV in arterial blood and venous blood?
8. What are the factors which influence PCV?
9. What is true haematocrit?
10. If you are given 1 ml of anticogulated blood to do only one investigation of maximum use, which should it be?
11. Classify anaemia based on blood indices.
12. Why does MCHC have an upper physiological limit?
13. What is the practical use of red cell indices in clinical haematology?

Student's Notes

Experiment 7: Determination of ESR

Aim

To find out the erythrocyte sedimentation rate (ESR) of the given sample of blood.

Principle

If blood containing an anticoagulant is allowed to stand in a tube placed vertically, the red cells settle down gradually to the bottom, since their specific gravity is greater than that of plasma. The rate at which the red cells settle down is noted.

Methods

Two methods are used to determine ESR:
1. Westergren's method
2. Wintrobe's method

WESTERGREN'S METHOD

Apparatus Required

A clean dry Westergren's tube, stand for the Westergren's tube sterile 3.8% sodium citrate solution. Westergren's tube is graduated from 0–200, 30 cm in length with an internal bore of 2.5 mm. It is open at both ends.

Procedure

1. 1.6 ml blood from the antecubital vein is diluted with 0.4 ml of 3.8% sodium citrate solution.
2. It is drawn into the Westergren's tube up to zero mark and fixed vertically in the Westergren's stand.
3. The cells settle down and the upper level of the cells is noted at the end of 1/2 hour and 1 hour.

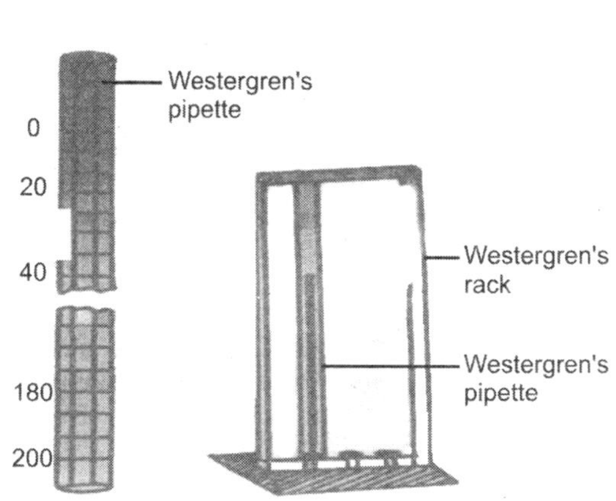

Fig. 7.1: Westergren's pipette and rack

Normal values:

Male 3–5 mm after 1 hr
Female and children 5–12 mm after 1 hr

WINTROBE'S METHOD

Apparatus Required

1. A clean dry Wintrobe's hematocrit tube. It is graduated in 1 mm to 100 mm and is open at the top and closed at the bottom. Its length is 11cm.
2. Wintrobe's hematocrit tube stand.
3. A test tube containing 2 mg of solid potassium oxalate and 3 mg of solid ammonium oxalate.
4. Pasteur pipette.
5. Spirit, sterile 2 ml syringe with needle, cotton and tourniquet.

Procedure

1. Blood drawn from the antecubital vein is mixed with anticoagulant and filled in the Wintrobe's tube up to zero mark with the help of Pasteur's pipette.
2. The tube is placed vertically in the stand.
3. The upper level of cells is noted at the end of 1/2 and 1 hour.

Normal values:

Males 0–9 mm after 1 hr
Females and children 0–20 mm after 1 hr

Precautions

1. The tube should be kept perfectly vertical.
2. Avoid air bubbles in the column of blood.
3. Blood should be used within 2 hours.
4. Blood showing any signs of coagulation or haemolysis should be rejected.
5. The test should be carried out at room temperature.
6. Avoid exposure to direct sunlight.
7. If excess of anticoagulant is used, it will alter the ESR value.

DISCUSSION

Erythrocyte Sedimentation Rate

This test measures the rate at which red cells settle spontaneously in a standing column of blood. This sedimentation process is divided into 3 stages for convenience.

Student's Notes

i. When, a column of blood stands undisturbed, there is a tendency of red cells to aggregate together in a peculiar 'pile of coins' arrangement called Rouleaux. This is the stage of aggregation.
ii. The aggregates get heavy and begin to fall to the bottom of the suspension. This is the stage of sedimentation called the stage of fall.
iii. The final phase is the stage of packing with the cells and aggregates low down due to increased cell concentration, crowding and packing.

Factors which Influence ESR

1. *Plasma protein:* This affects the stage of rouleaux formation. Fibrinogen and globulin increase rouleaux formation opposite to albumin which has a retarding effect. When rouleaux formation increases, ESR increases.
   In conditions where there is an increase in fibrinogen or globulin, ESR is increased. Examples are chronic infections like TB and systemic inflammatory disorders like rheumatoid arthritis. All these conditions have tissue injury and immune reactions, both, leading to high levels of fibrinogen and globulins (all antibodies are globulins).
2. *Red cell count:* The total number of red cells also affects ESR; but not to such an extent as the plasma proteins. In anaemia, there is more space between the red cells and it is easier for them to fall and for the displaced plasma to rise than when the cells are relatively more crowded in conditions like polycythemia. Therefore an ESR in a severely anaemic person should be given guarded consideration because, anaemia will increase ESR more.

Significance of ESR in Disease

1. The increase in ESR is not diagnostic of any disease but it has only prognostic value.
2. It only indicates increase in fibrinogen/globulin levels, as would happen in any tissue injury.
3. The ESR is used to check the progress of the patient. As the patient improves, the ESR tends to fall. If the patient's condition is getting worse, the ESR tends to rise.

Physiological Variations

Increased

1. Pregnancy
2. Menstruation
3. Parturition.

Decreased

Very rare in newborn babies.

Pathological Variations

Increased

1. Rheumatic fever.
2. Tuberculosis.
3. Malignancy.
4. Anaemia.

Decreased

1. Polycythemia.
2. Congenital absence of fibrinogen.
3. Congenital spherocytosis.
4. Allergic conditions.

Factors affecting ESR

1. *Specific gravity:* Corpuscles of 'high' specific gravity settle down in plasma of low specific gravity.
2. Lowered viscosity of plasma increases ESR.
3. *Size of RBC:* Increased RBC size leads to increased ESR.
4. Clumping of cells increases ESR.
5. Spherocytes reduce ESR due to prevention of rouleaux formation.
6. Increase of temperatures leads to increase in ESR.
7. High RBC count decreases ESR.
8. Increase in plasma lecithin decreases ESR.
9. Increase in fibrinogen increases ESR. Increase in albumin decreases it.

Result

The erythrocyte sedimentation rate of the given subject is..........

QUESTIONS

1. Mention some common infections and inflammatory disorders which show increase in ESR. What is the cause of this increase?
2. In multiple myeloma, what is the reason for an increased ESR?
3. What is the importance of monitoring the ESR in a patient with tuberculosis?
4. What is the only normal condition in which ESR is decreased?
5. Compare the effects of anaemia and polycythemia on the ESR?
6. What are the methods by which ESR can be determined?
7. What are the factors affecting ESR?
8. What is the clinical significance of this investigation?

Student's Notes

9. What is the normal ESR value in Westergren's method?
10. What is the normal ESR value in Wintrobe's method?
11. Mention some pathological conditions which decrease ESR.
12. What is the advantage of using the double oxalate mixture in Wintrobe's method? Can we use any other anticoagulants?
13. Why the normal values of ESR are more with Wintrobe's method as compared to Westergren's?
14. Why ESR reading is taken normally after one hour?

Student's Notes

Experiment 8: Total Leucocyte Count

Aim

To enumerate the white blood cells in 1 mm^3 of blood.

Principle

The blood is diluted with a diluting fluid which destroys the red blood corpuscles and stains the nuclei of the white blood cells. The leucocytes are then counted in a haemocytometer and their number in undiluted blood is calculated.

Apparatus Required

Microscope, haemocytometer, WBC pipette, Turk's fluid, cover slip, disposable lancet, cotton and spirit.

Composition of Turk's Fluid

Glacial acetic acid	1.5 ml (or) 2 ml
Gentian violet	1 ml
Distilled water	100 ml

Glacial acetic acid destroys RBC; gentian violet colours the nuclei of WBC.

Procedure

i. *Filling the pipette and diluting the blood sample:* Clean the finger tip with spirit and prick it with a sterile lancet. The first drop of blood is discarded as it contains tissue fluid. Allow a good sized drop to form and draw blood up to 0.5 in the WBC pipette. Suck the Turk's fluid up to the mark 11. Hold the pipette horizontally and roll it between the palms to ensure thorough mixing.

ii. *Charging the chamber:* Place the cover slip over the chamber. Place the chamber on the microscope stage. Roll the pipette again before charging. Discard the first two or three drops of fluid as the stem of the pipette is filled only with diluting fluid and has no blood at all.

Allow a moderate size drop of diluted blood to form at the tip of the pipette. Hold the pipette at an angle of 45° and make the drop to touch the slide and the cover slip. The fluid will run into the capillary space to fill it. The fluid should not run into the trenches. There should be no air bubbles in the chamber. After charging allow the fluid then to settle for 2–3 minutes before actual counting is begun.

iii. *Counting the cells:* Focus the WBC area under low power and ensure that there is no air bubble. The cells lying on the upper horizontal and left vertical lines should be counted along with those lying within the square under consideration. Count the cells in 4 large corner squares and enter in the observation table.

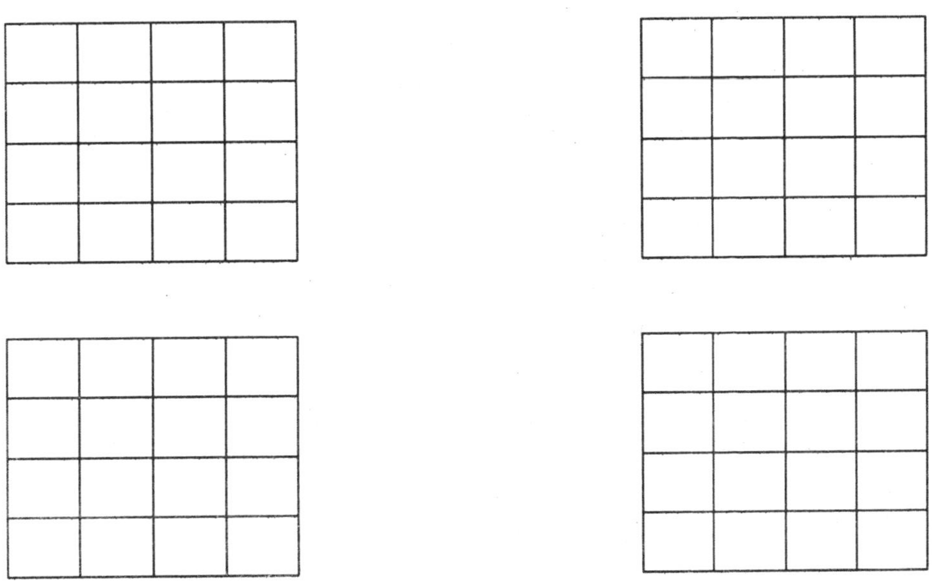

Total no of cells in 64 small squares =

Student's Notes

Precautions

1. There should be no air bubble in the column of the blood.
2. The cells should be evenly distributed.

Calculation

No of cells in four large WBC square	= x
No of cells in one WBC square	= x/4
Side of 1 WBC square	= 1 mm
Area of 1 WBC square	= 1 mm^2
Depth of chamber	= 1/10 mm
Volume of fluid present over 1 WBC square	= 1/10 mm^3
No of cells in 1/10 cu mm of diluted blood	= x/4
No of cells in 1 cu mm of diluted blood	= x/4 × 10
Dilution factor	= 1:20
No of cells in 1 cu mm of undiluted blood	= x/4 × 10 × 20
	= 50x

DISCUSSION

(Normal range of WBC is 4000–11000 cu mm in one) Total leucocytes count shows variation under certain physiological and pathological conditions.

Leucocytosis (increase in WBC Count)

Physiological Conditions

i. Age
   a. Newborn will always have an increased count.
   b. Childhood, pregnancy and delivery shows increased count.
   c. There is no significant change in old age compared to adult values.

ii. Females during pregnancy and parturition.

iii. Stress like severe exercise, severe pain, and excitation.

iv. Diurnal variation: WBC count may vary from hour to hour. Highest count in evening and lowest count in morning).

v. Digestive leucocytosis (after digestion).

vi. Injection of adrenaline.

Pathological Conditions

a. *Acute pyogenic infections:* For example, pneumonia, appendicitis and tonsillitis.
b. *Leukaemia (abnormal increase with immature cells):* Count may go up to 1,00,000 to 3, 00,000 per cu mm.
c. Acute haemorrhage.
d. Tissue damage resulting from burns, operations, myocardial infarction.
e. Malignant neoplasms.
f. Metabolic disorder—For example, gout, diabetic acidosis

Leucopenia (decrease in WBC count)

Physiological Conditions

Rare but sometimes due to:

1. Exposure to cold
2. Aspirin.

Pathological Conditions

a. Infection—typhoid.
b. Starvation—malnutrition.
c. Viral infections—measles, chickenpox, influenza, rubella
d. Drugs—antimetabolites, antimicrobials (sulphonamides, chloramphenicol).
e. Haematological disorders—aplastic anaemia, pernicious anaemia, irradiation).

QUESTIONS

1. Is this a routine test? What is the usefulness of this test?
2. What other test has to be done with total count to make it more meaningful?
3. Why should you destroy the RBCs while doing WBC count?
4. What is the normal range of total WBC count? List 3 important physiological variations?

Student's Notes

Experiment 9: Differential Count of White Blood Cells

Aim

To enumerate the different types of white blood cells in the given subject.

Apparatus Required

Microscope, clean dry grease free glass slides with even edges, a drop bottle containing distilled water, a drop bottle containing Leishman's stain, cedar wood oil, staining rack, lancet, cotton, spirit.

Composition of Leishman's Stain

Eosin: An acidic dye which stains the basic protoplasmic material.

Methylene blue: A basic dye which stains the acidic nuclear chromatin.

Acetone free methyl alcohol: To fix the smear to the slide. Acetone being a strong lipid solvent it tends to damage the cell membrane. The stain is prepared by dissolving 750 mg of Leishman's powder in 500 ml of acetone free methyl alcohol.

Procedure Preparation of Blood Film

1. The finger is cleaned and pricked with a sterile lancet.
2. The first drop of blood is discarded.
3. A clean glass slide is touched to the newly formed drop of blood 1 cm away from the edge.
4. The slide is placed on the table so that the blood drop is on the right side. It is supported with the left hand and the second slide (spreader) is held along its long edges with the right hand at an angle 45°.

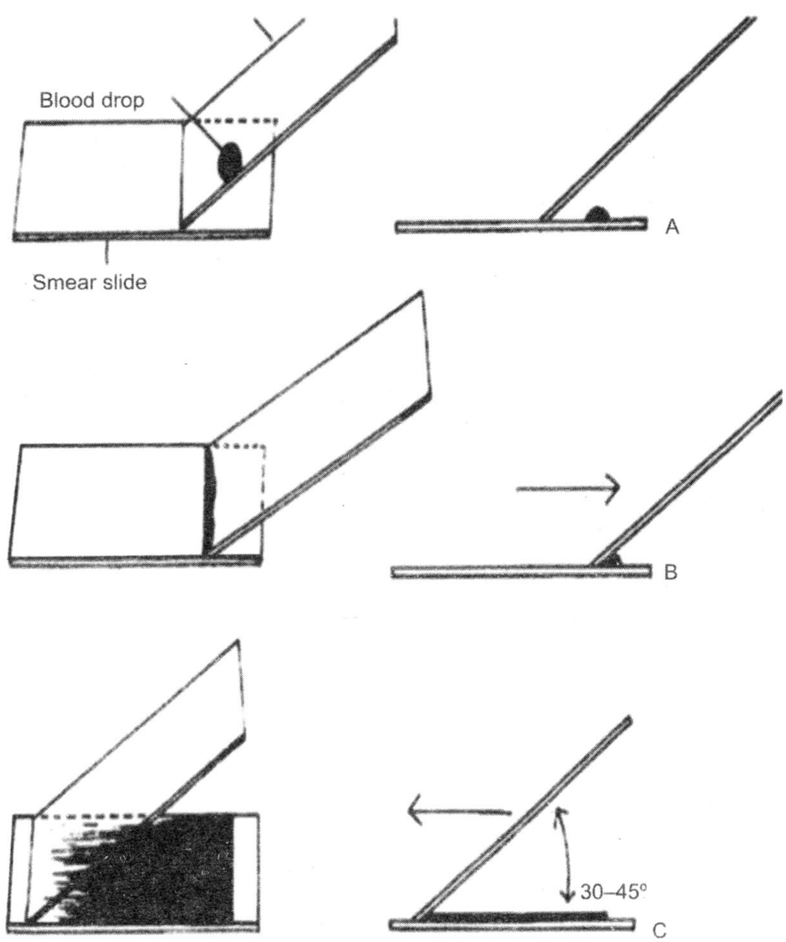

Fig. 9.1

5. The smooth narrow edge of the spreader slide is placed in front of the blood drop and drawn back to touch the drop which then spreads along the edge of the spreader slide evenly. The spreader slide is pushed towards the left and towards left by a quick uniform motion with a light but even pressure. The blood follows along the spreader slide to form a blood film. It is dried quickly by waving in the air.

Staining the Blood Film

The blood smear is placed on the staining rack. Leishman's stain is added drop by drop till the entire film is covered by the stain. The numbers of drops added are counted (usually 8–10 drops). The undiluted stain is allowed to act for 2 minutes. It should not be allowed to dry up. The cells are fixed in these 2 minutes. Then, double the number of distilled water drops is added to dilute the stain. It is mixed by gently blowing through a pipette. The actual staining occurs now only. The stain should not be allowed to dry. After 7 minutes, the stain is drained off. The slide is washed in a gentle stream of running tap water until the film turns pink. The slide is kept in a vertical position to drain and dry. Thick uneven smears should be discarded. It is preferable to make 3-4 smears. The best stained film should be selected for microscopic examination. A good smear should:

1. Be buff coloured
2. Be uniform
3. Be broader at the head and taper off into a tail
4. Occupy the middle third of the slide leaving a margin of about 5 mm along the edges.
5. Have no longitudinal or transverse striations or windows.
6. Have no stained granules or precipitates.
7. Have discrete red cells without overlapping each other.

Microscopic Examination

The microscope is adjusted for oil immersion lens. The condenser is raised, the diaphragm is completely opened and the plane mirror is used. Two drops of cedar wood oil are placed near the head end. The oil immersion objective lens is made to touch the oil by viewing from the side. The fine adjustment screw is adjusted till the cells are brought into focus.

Hundred squares are drawn for recording the cell count. The white blood cells are identified and entered using the letter N for neutrophil, E for eosinophil, B for basophil, L for lymphocyte and M for monocyte. The slide is slowly moved towards the tail end and the cells are counted. The slide is then shifted up and moved in the opposite direction. This pattern of movement of the slide (zigzag pattern) takes into consideration all the parts of the film and ensures that a cell is not counted more than once.

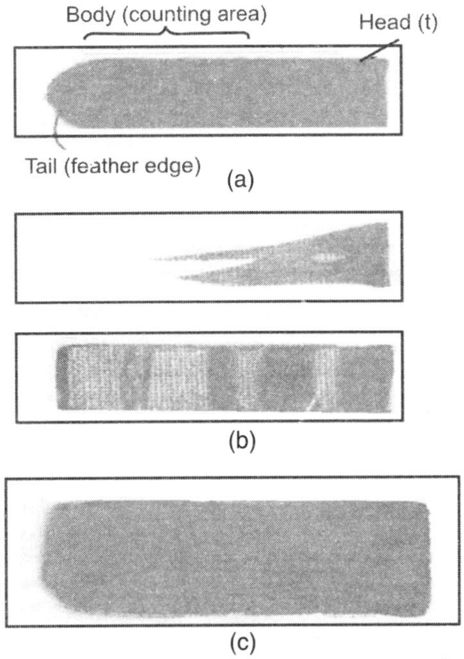

Fig. 9.2: Good (a) and bad (b, c) smears

Hundred white cells are identified and entered. The number of each type of white blood cell is counted and expressed in percentage.

Identification of the Cells

A leukocyte is identified from its size, the nucleus and the cytoplasm.

Size

The size of the white cell is assessed by comparing it to that of the red cells (7.2). If the white cell is as big as the red cell, it probably is a small lymphocyte. If the cell is twice as big as the red cell, it may be a granulocyte or a large lymphocyte. If the cell is about 2. 1/2 to 3 times, then it is possibly a monocyte.

Nucleus

The following characters of the nucleus must be observed:

a. Whether it appears as a single mass or lobed
b. If single, whether the shape is round-, oval- or kidney-shaped
c. Whether partially or completely fills the cell.

A small cell with a single round or oval nucleus may be a small lymphocyte. A bigger cell with distinct

Student's Notes

nuclear lobes joined by chromatin strands should be a granulocyte. A big cell with a kidney-shaped nucleus is a monocyte. The nucleus in a lymphocyte completely fills the cells.

Cytoplasm

a. The amount of cytoplasm in relation to the size of the nucleus is noted.
b. The presence of visible granules and their nature is observed.

A small cell with a thin crescent of cytoplasm is a small lymphocyte. A bigger cell with a rim of cytoplasm all around is a large lymphocyte. A big cell with large amount of clear cytoplasm in relation to the nucleus is a monocyte.

If a granulocyte has fine neutral granules of light violet colour, the cell is a neutrophil. If the granules are coarse and orange or red coloured, the cell is an eosinophil. In a basophil, the granules are large, coarse and deep blue in colour. It is the smallest of all granulocytes.

Results

Neutrophils	%
Eosinophils	%
Basophils	%
Lymphocytes	%
Monocytes	%

DISCUSSION

The percentage of the different types of white blood cells is called the differential count. It is done to find out if there is an increase or decrease in a particular type of leukocyte. But it shows only a relative increase or decrease of the cell type with a corresponding change in the other cell types. Absolute values are more significant relative value.

Normal Count

Neutrophils	50–70%
Eosinophils	1–4%
Basophils	0–1%
Lymphocytes	20–40%
Monocytes	2–8%

Causes

Neutrophilia

It is an increase in the number of neutrophils:

1. Acute pyogenic infection such as tonsillitis, appendicitis, pneumonia
2. Tissue necrosis as in myocardial infarction
3. Following haemorrhage
4. Trauma, postoperative burns
5. Haemolysis
6. Malignant neoplasm
7. Metabolic disorders like gout, diabetic acidosis, uremia
8. Drugs such as glucocorticoids, adrenaline, digitalis, phenacetin
9. Poisoning with lead, mercury, insect venom.
10. Physiological-exercise, stress, after meals, pregnancy and parturition.

Neutropenia

Neutropenia is decrease in the number of neutrophils:

1. Typhoid and paratyphoid fever, kala azar
2. Viral infection
3. Depression of bone marrow due to irradiation,

Cell type	*Size*	*Nucleus*	*Cytoplasm*
Granulocyte			
Neutrophil	10–14 μm	2–6 lobes connected by chromatin	Fine light violet coloured granules
Eosinophil	10–14 μm	Bicobed connected by a chromatin strand (spectacle-shaped)	Coarse orange to brick red granules.
Basophil	10–14 μm	Irregular may be bilobed or S-shaped. Not seen clearly as it is obscured by the granules.	Coarse deep blue granules completely filling the cell.
Agranulocytes			
Lymphocyte			
Small	8–10 μm	Large-round nucleus completely, filling the cell, stains deep blue.	Thin crescent of pale blue cytoplasm. No granules seen
Large	10–15 μm	Large round or indented nucleus, stains deep blue	Thin rim of pale blue cytoplasm all around. No granules seen
Monocyte	16–24 μm	Large, placed centrally, kidney-shaped nucleus	Large amount of pale grey blue cytoplasm. No granules seen.

Student's Notes

Draw a neat diagram of

Neutrophil

Eosinophil

Basophil

Lymphocyte

Monocyte

4. Drugs such as chloramphenicol
5. Autoimmune diseases.

Eosinophilia

Increase in the number of eosinophils:

1. Allergic conditions like asthma, hay fever, urticaria
2. Parasitic infestations—such as trichinosis, schistosomiasis, hookworm infestation.
3. Tropical eosinophilia
4. Skin diseases like eczema
5. Loeffler's syndrome
6. Collagen disorders
7. Chronic myeloid leukaemia
8. Hodgkin's disease.

Eosinopenia

Decrease in the number of eosinophils:

1. Administration of ACTH and glucocorticoids
2. Stress
3. Cushing's syndrome
4. Acute pyogenic infections.

Basophilia

Increase in the number of basophils:

1. Viral infections such as smallpox and chickenpox
2. Allergic disease
3. Chronic myeloid leukaemia and polycythemia vera.

Basopenia

Decrease in the number of basophils:

1. Acute pyogenic infection
2. Glucocorticoid treatment.

Monocytosis

Increase in the number of monocytes:

1. Chronic infection like tuberculosis, syphilis, subacute bacterial endocarditis, brucellosis
2. Protozoal infections like malaria, kala azar
3. Infectious mononucleosis
4. Monocytic leukaemia and multiple myeloma
5. Collagen diseases
6. Granulomatous diseases like sarcoidosis,ulcerative colitis.

Monocytopenia

Decrease in the number of monocytes occurs rarely in:

1. Bone marrow failure
2. Aplastic anaemia
3. Septicaemia

Student's Notes

Lymphocytosis

Increase in the number of lymphocytes:

1. Infants and young children(relative lymphocytosis)
2. Whooping cough, diphtheria
3. Chronic infections like TB, syphilis and malaria
4. Viral infection like chickenpox
5. Lymphocytic leukaemia
6. Autoimmune diseases.

Lymphocytopenia

Decrease in the number of lymphocytes:

1. Steroid therapy
2. Acute infections and illnesses
3. Hodgkin's disease
4. Bone marrow failure.

QUESTIONS

1. What is the purpose of methyl alcohol in Leishman's stain?
2. What is the pH of the buffered water that is used?
3. Give the normal differential count. What are the physiological variations?
4. Explain the terms:
   a. Neutrophilia and
   b. Neutropenia and list conditions where it occurs.
5. What are the terms which refer to:
   a. Increase and
   b. Decrease in the lymphocyte count?
   Name two conditions in which each occurs.
6. What is monocytosis? When does it occur?
7. What is the composition of Leishman's stain? What are the functions of each component?
8. Name some conditions where eosinophils and neutrophils increase in number.
9. Which WBC has got the phagocytic function?
10. What is the function of lymphocytes in the body?
11. What are the special features of monocytes? How will you differentiate monocytes from large lymphocytes?
12. How do you differentiate a bilobed eosinophil from a neutrophils?
13. What are microscopic adjustments you will do before starting the experiment ?
14. Why methyl alcohol should be acetone free?

Student's Notes

Experiment 10: Absolute Eosinophil Count

Aim

To estimate the absolute eosinophil count of the given sample of blood.

Apparatus Required

Haemocytometer, microscope, cotton, spirit, sterile needle or lancet, Pilot's fluid.

Pilot's Fluid

Phloxine 1% aqueous	10 ml
Propylene glycol	50 ml
Distilled water	40 ml
Sodium carbonates 10%	1 ml

Phloxine stains the granules of the eosinophils. Propylene glycol and distilled water lyses the RBCs. Sodium carbonate accelerates staining.

Dunger's fluid may also be used to stain the eosinophil. It contains:

Eosin	0.01 g
Acetone	10 ml

Distilled water to make up to 100 ml

This Dunger's fluid is used in this experiment.

Procedure

1. After sterilising the finger, obtain a drop of blood by finger puncture.
2. Draw blood up to mark 1 in the WBC pipette and immediately immerse into the diluting fluid and draw the fluid up to mark 11.
3. Mix the fluid well by rolling the pipette in the palm.
4. Keep it aside for 15 minutes for adequate staining of the cells.
5. Discard the fluid in the stem of the pipette and charge the counting chamber.

Total no of cells in 9 big squares =

6. Count the cells (eosinophils alone are stained) in all 9 large squares.

Calculation

Number of cells in 9 large squares	= X
Number of cells in one large square	= X/9
Side of one large square	= 1 mm
Area of one large square	= 1 × 1 = 1 sq.mm
Depth of chamber	= 1/10 mm
Volume over one large square	= IX 1/10 cu mm
No of cells in 1/10 cu mm of diluted blood	= X/9
No of cells in 1 cu mm of diluted blood	= X/9 × 10
Dilution factor	= 1:10
No of cells in 1 cu mm of undiluted blood	= X/9 × 10 × 10
	$= \frac{100X}{9}$

Precautions

Same as those observed for RBC and WBC count.

Normal value: 40 to 440 cells/mm^3.

Variations

Eosinophilia (increase in eosinophil count) is seen in:

1. Allergic disorder:
   - Bronchial asthma
   - Hay fever
   - Urticaria due to drug sensitivity especially
   - Sulphonamides and aspirin
2. Skin diseases: For example, pemphigus
3. Parasitic infestations especially parasites that invade the tissues, e.g. trichinosis, echinococcus disease.
4. Tropical eosinophilia
5. Loeffler's syndrome
6. Certain diseases of hemopoietic system, e.g. polycythemia vera, Hodgekin's disease, pernicious anaemia.
7. Following irradiation
8. Rheumatoid arthritis
9. Sarcoidosis
10. Idiopathic

Student's Notes

Eosinopenia (decrease in eosinophil count) in seen:

1. Following corticosteroid therapy
2. Following ACTH injection
3. During neutrophilia
4. Emotional stress

QUESTIONS

1. What is the normal total eosinophil count?
2. Mention the functions of eosinophils.
3. Name the conditions in which there is an increase in the absolute eosinophil count?
4. Name the hormone which causes a lowering of eosinophil count?
5. What is the appearance of an eosinophil in a stained smear? What do the granules contain?
6. What is the significance of doing absolute eosinophil count?
7. What is major basic protein? What is its role?
8. Mention the composition of Dunger's fluid.
9. With a diagram show the morphology of eosinophils.
10. What is the dilution used in eosinophil count?
11. What is the chemotactic factor for eosinophil?
12. How eosinophils combat infestation by worms?
13. Name the chemicals in the eosinophil granules.

Experiment 11: Determination of Bleeding Time and Clotting Time

BLEEDING TIME

Aim

To determine the bleeding time of the given subject by Duke's method.

Apparatus Required

Filter paper, stop clock, lancet, cotton, spirit.

Procedure

The tip of the left ring finger is pricked with aseptic precautions (3–4 mm). The blood should flow freely without squeezing. The time of puncture is noted. With a filter paper, the blood is gently blotted every 30 seconds. The successive blots become smaller. This procedure is repeated until no blot appears on the filter paper. The time is noted again. The number of blots on the paper is counted. Number of blots × 30 seconds will be the bleeding time.

Discussion

Bleeding time is the time interval between the skin puncture and the cessation of bleeding—the time in minutes which it takes for a standardized skin wound to stop bleeding. Significance: Cessation of bleeding from a small wound as that inflicted during this procedure can be affected by vascular spasm and formation of platelet plugs. This test therefore measures the capillary and platelet functions in haemostasis.
Normal: 1–5 minutes (by Duke's method).

Factors which affect the Bleeding Time

1. Size and nature of the injury
2. Condition of the vessel wall
3. Number of platelets.

Conditions where Bleeding Time is Prolonged

1. Decrease in the number of platelets—thrombocytopenic purpura
2. Functional platelet defect:
   a. Drugs like aspirin, penicillin
   b. von Willebrand's disease
   c. Uraemia, cirrhosis, leukaemia
3. Vessel wall defects:
   a. Prolonged treatment with corticosteroids
   b. Allergic purpuras
   c. Infections with haemolytic streptococci, bacterial endocarditis
   d. Deficiency of vitamin C
   e. Senile purpura.

Other Methods

1. In Duke's mehtod, the edge of the ear lobe can also be used
2. *Ivy's method:* The cuff of the BP apparatus is applied to the upper arm and the pressure is raised to 40 mm Hg.The front of the fore arm is used. The normal bleeding time by this method is up to 9 min.
3. The finger is pricked and dipped in a beaker containing normal saline at 37°C. The blood drops will be seen falling to the bottom of the beaker in a continuous slow stream. The time is noted when the bleeding stops.
4. Capillary fragility test of HESS or tourniquet test. The bleeding time may be performed by Duke's method or Ivy's method; Ivy's method is a recommended method, but in this lab, we follow Duke's method for the sake of convenience.

Result

The bleeding time of the given subject is..........

CLOTTING TIME

Aim

To determine the clotting time of the given subject by Wright's method.

Apparatus Required

Capillary glass tube 15 cm long with a bore of 0.8 mm, stop clock, lancet, cotton, spirit.

Procedure

The tip of the left ring finger is pricked under aseptic precautions and the time of puncture is noted. The prick must be deep enough to allow free flow of blood without squeezing.

The blood is drawn into the capillary tube by dipping one end of the tube in the blood drop. The blood fills the tube by capillary action. After 2 minutes, a small bit of the tube is broken every 30 seconds until a fine thread of fibrin appears between the broken ends. The time is again noted and the interval between the prick and the appearance of fibrin threads gives the clotting time.

Student's Notes

Discussion

Clotting time is the time interval between the skin puncture and formation of fibrin thread. Significance: The clotting time is generally not affected by deficiency of platelets as only few platelets are required to provide enough platelet factor 3 for normal coagulation. This test assesses the intrinsic and common pathways of coagulation because the trigger for coagulation in this test is the surface activation of blood that comes into contact with the glass surface of the test tube (therefore for comparability, we should use standard size tubes and constant blood volumes so that the same amount of surface activation occur each time).
Normal: 2–8 minutes.

Conditions where Clotting Time is Prolonged

1. Haemophilia (bleeding time is normal)
2. Christmas disease
3. Afibrinogenemia
4. Vitamin K deficiency
5. Liver disease
6. Anticoagulant therapy
7. Newborn baby.

OTHER METHODS

1. *Lee and white method:* 1 ml of blood is placed in 8 mm diameter tube. The tube is tilted at definite time intervals until there is no displacement of fluid blood, when the tube is inverted.
2. *Drop method:* A drop of blood is placed on a glass slide. Clotting is indicated by the absence of any change in the shape of the drop when the slide is held vertical.

Lee and White's method is the most accurate and recommended method. But since it involves larger quantities of blood and venous sampling, this method will 'only be demonstrated to you. For individual exercises you will do the Wright's capillary tube method.

Result

The clotting time of the given subject is.........

Tests of Hemostasis

The first line tests for each of the following mechanisms of haemostasis are:

1. Vascular integrity—bleeding time
2. Platelet function—bleeding time and platelet count
3. Coagulation mechanism – Clotting count
   – PTT
   – One stage prothrombin time fibrinogen assay

In this course, you will learn to perform the following tests of haemostasis.

1. Bleeding time
2. Clotting time
3. Platelet count.

QUESTIONS

1. What happens to bleeding time in each of the following disorders of haemostasis and why?
   a. Thrombocytopenia
   b. von Willebrand's disease
   c. Haemophilia
   d. Thrombasthenia
   e. Pseudoxanthoma elastican (vascular discover)
   f. Scurvy.
   g. A. fibrinogenemia
2. List 4 conditions where clotting time is increased.
3. What happens to the following tests of haemostasis in each of the following conditions?

	Platelet count	*Bleeding time*	*Clotting time*
Thrombocytopenia			
Haemophilia			
Obstructive jaundice			
Heparin therapy			
von Willebrand's disease			
Thrombasthenia			

4. What is the normal platelet count?
5. What are the functions of platelets?
6. Name two conditions where platelet counts may be abnormally
   a. High b. Low
7. What are the clinical effects of a low platelet count?
8. Explain the term thrombasthenia. What is its clinical significance?
9. Name the different methods by which you can determine clotting time.
10. Name the diseases where bleeding time and clotting time are altered; explain briefly the reasons for the alterations.
11. Why the bleeding time is normally shorter than clotting lime?
12. What is haemostasis? Name the different mechanisms involved in it.
13. What is the natural anticoagulant present in the human body?

Student's Notes

14. Name some of the anticoagulants used clinically.
15. What is thrombosis?
16. What is an embolus?
17. Enumerate the various coagulation factors.
18. What is prothrombin time and what is its significance?
19. Name some other tests used in coagulation disorders.

Student's Notes

Experiment 12: Blood Grouping

Synonym: Blood typing

Introduction: It is essential to know the blood group of a person, if he is encountered by anyone of the following circumstances.

1. Blood transfusions
2. Paternity disputes
3. Medicolegal problems
4. Organ transplantation.

Transplantations

The current system of blood grouping was discovered by Land Steiner in 1900 and is known as the Land Steiner's ABO system.

Principle

The RBCs contain a series of antigens known as agglutinogens on their cell membrane while the plasma contains antibodies known as agglutinins. To find out a person's blood group, the RBCs are made to react with antisera containing known agglutinins. The slide is then observed for the presence or absence of agglutination and haemolysis of RBC. This can be done with the naked eye but is ideally done by viewing the slide under the microscope.

Apparatus and Reagents Required

1. Sterile lancet
2. Cotton swab
3. Alcohol
4. Glass dropper
5. Toothpicks
6. Microscope
7. Porcelain tile
8. 3.8% sodium citrate in normal saline
9. Abti-A serum
10. Anti-B serum
11. Anti-D serum.

Note: Anti-A serum is tinted blue and anti-B serum is tinted yellow.

Procedure

With a glass marking pencil, the porcelain tile is divided into 3 portions. Under aseptic conditions, the subject whose blood group is to be determined is asked to stick out his finger which is pricked and 3–4 drops of blood is then obtained. Following this the blood is diluted with 1 ml of 3.8% sodium citrate in normal saline taken in a test tube. A drop of anti-A, anti-B and anti-D sera is placed on each of the 3 portions on the tile. Now 1 drop of the diluted blood is put on each of the 3 portions containing the sera. This is mixed with 3 separate toothpicks. After 10–15 minutes, each portion is examined for clumping and agglutination first with the naked eye and then under the microscope.

Observation and Results

If any agglutination occurs, it is usually visible to the naked eye as dark red clumps of different sizes. The presence or absence of agglutination indicates the blood group of the subject as shown in the Table 12.1.

Table 12.1

Agglutination		Subject's blood group
With anti-A serum present	*With anti-B serum absent*	
Present	Absent	A
Absent	Present	B
Present	Present	AB
Absent	Absent	0

Conclusion: Having determined the subject's blood group his Rh typing can be determined in a similar fashion using anti-Rh serum (Anti-D serum).

Result

The blood group of the given blood sample is.........

QUESTIONS

1. The approximate percentages of people in each of these blood groups in South India is as follows: 0 group....... 45%, B group........ 30%, A group..... 20%, AB group......... 5%. Ascertain the blood group of a large part of your class as possible and calculate the percentages. How do these values vary compared to those of the general population?
2. What is your blood group? Illustrate your observations.
3. How are the A and B antigens inherited?
4. What is the practical importance of blood grouping?
5. What is a transfusion reaction? Differentiate between a major and a minor transfusion reaction.

Student's Notes

6. Mention another important system of blood grouping. How does the ABO system differ from this system of grouping? Give the clinical importance of this system.
7. What is Landsteiner's law?
8. Name the different types of blood groups you know.
9. What is the main difference between the ABO group and the Rh factor?
10. What is cross-matching?
11. What are the uses of blood groups?
12. What is Bombay blood group?
13. Why is blood group '0' known as universal donor?
14. What is the importance of MN group?
15. What is the composition of ACD mixture?
16. Which preservative (anticoagulant) is used for storing blood?
17. What is the difference between rouleaux formation and aglutination?

Student's Notes

Experiment 13: Osmotic Fragility of Red Blood Cells

Aim

To determine the osmotic fragility of red blood cells.

Apparatus Required

Ten clean test tubes, test tube rack, disposable syringe with needle, spirit swab, dropper bottle, 3.8% sodium citrate and saline solutions of following concentrations—0.70%. 0.65%, 0.60%, 0.55%, 0.50%. 0.45%, 0.40%, 0.35%, and 0.30%.

Preparation of Sodium Chloride Solutions

A 1% stock solution is prepared by dissolving 1 gm of NaCl in 100 ml of distilled water. To make 0.70% NaCl 70 ml of stock solution is diluted with 30 ml of distilled water. To make 0.65% NaCl: 65 ml of stock solution is diluted with 35 ml of distilled water. Thus sodium chloride solution of different concentrations is prepared accordingly.

Procedure

1. Ten test tubes containing sodium chloride solutions of varying concentration from 0.70% to 0.30% are placed in a test tube rack.
2. The blood drawn intravenously is mixed with the anticoagulant in the beaker.
3. With the help of a dropper, a drop of blood is added into each of the test tube and mixed thoroughly by inverting the tubes several times.
4. Alternatively a finger is pricked and a drop of blood is squeezed into each of the test tube.
5. The tubes are allowed to stand for one hour.
6. At the end of the hour, the test tube where haemolysis has just begun (supernatant fluid just becomes red) and the test tube where haemolysis is incomplete (whole solution is uniformly red) are noted.

Discussion

Fluid diffuses through the membrane into the red blood cells when it is placed in hypotonic solution. The movement of fluid depends on the surface area of the membrane. The cells get distended and lysed. Normal red blood cells commence lysing at 0.48% saline and end or complete at 0.34% saline solution.

Osmotic fragility is increased in the following conditions:

1. Hereditary spherocytosis
2. Venous blood cells are more fragile than arterial blood cells
3. Stored blood
4. Increased intracellular osmotic pressure.

Osmotic resistance (decreased fragility) is seen in the following conditions.

1. Thalassemia
2. Sickle cell anaemia
3. Disorders in which leptocytes including 'target' cells are found.

Principle of this Experiment

This is a quantitative experiment assessing the degree of fragility of red blood cells. A series of test tubes of various concentrations of NaCl solutions are taken and a drop of blood is added to each of them. The tubes at which haemolysis begins and is complete are noted and reported.

Discussion

Osmosis is the process which governs transport of solvent between two solutions separated by a membrane which is relatively impermeable to the solute.When an RBC is placed in:

1. A solution of 0.9% saline, no exchange of water takes place. This solution is said to be isotonic with the interior of the RBC.
2. Dilute NaCl solution, (concentration of NaCl less than 0.9%) water enters the cell. This solution is said to be hypotonic with respect to the interior of the RBC.
3. Concentrated NaCl solution, (concentration of NaCl more than 0.9%) water leaves the cell. This solution is said to be hypertonic with respect to the interior of the RBC.

As the RBC is a biconcave disc, when placed in hypotonic solution it is able to take up water till it attains the spherical shape. If the tonicity of the solution is very low then the cell is unable to contain the excess inflow of water and it bursts (hemolysis). On the other hand, when the cell is placed in a highly concentrated NaCl solution, water leaves the cell and the cell shrinks. (crenation). On placing the cell in an isotonic solution, no change occurs.

Significance

1. In normal healthy individuals, osmotic fragility of RBCs begins at 0.48% NaCl and ends at 0.34% NaCl solution.

Student's Notes

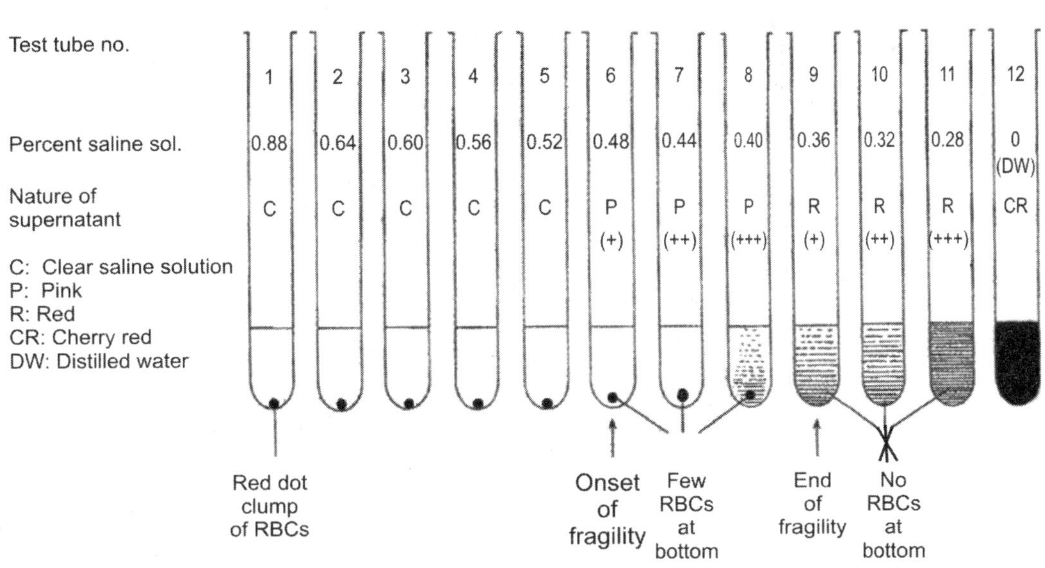

Fig. 13.1: Unit 1: Haematology

2. RBC's osmotic fragility increases when it becomes spherical, e.g. in spherocytosis (independent of the cause). It begins at 0.7% NaCl and ends at 0.45% NaCl solution.
3. RBC's osmotic fragility is decreased when it becomes slender, e.g. in iron deficiency anaemia and in thalassaemia. It begins at 0.36% NaCl and ends at 0.24% NaCl solution.

Result

Haemolysis begins at ....% saline and ends at ....% saline.

QUESTIONS

1. Would you say the fragility is increased or decreased in the following situations?
   a. Haemolysis begins at 0.55 g% and is complete at 0.45 g%
   b. Haemolysis beings at 0.3 g% and is completed at 0.25 g%.
2. Name one condition where fragility is increased and say why?
3. Name one condition where fragility is decreased.
4. Name one other aetiology where fragility is increased in the RBC.
5. What is the difference between isotonic and iso-osmotic solutions?
6. Define the terms haemolysis and crenation: When do they occur?
7. Name some haemolytic agents.
8. What is mechanical fragility and how is it tested?
9. Do all the normal RBCs present in the given sample of blood have the same osmotic fragility to hypotonic solutions?
10. What happens to the osmotic fragility of RBCs in an individual after splenectomy?
11. Define the terms osmosis and osmotic pressure. How much osmotic pressure is exerted by the blood and what is its importance in the body?
12. Explain the mechanism of haemolysis of RBCs of the body?

Student's Notes

Experiment 14: Specific Gravity of Blood

Aim

To determine the specific gravity of the given sample of blood by Van Slyke's falling drop method.

Principle

The specific gravity of blood is determined by comparing the specific gravity of a drop of blood with that of solutions of known specific gravity.

Apparatus and Reagent

1. Stock solutions of copper sulphate of 1.1 specific gravity. It is prepared by dissolving 170 g of blue vitriol ($CuSO_4+5H_2O$) in 1.0024 litres of distilled water.
2. Distilled water
3. 4 test tubes
4. Clean dry sterilised syringe with needle
5. Cotton and rectified spirit.

Preparation of Solution

Two miscible liquids of known but different specific gravity (copper sulphate and water) are mixed in varying proportions.

The stock solution of $CuSO_4$ with specific gravity 1.100 and distilled water with specific gravity 1.000 are mixed in varying proportions to give standard solutions of $CuSO_4$ with specific gravity varying from 1.049 to 1.064.

Advantages of copper sulphate solution:

1. It is cheap and easily available
2. It is not hygroscopic
3. It is not volatile or inflammable.
4. It can be repeatedly used.
5. The temperature coefficient of expansion of CuSO4 solution and blood are equal and platelet count and no correction for temperature is required.

Other solutions used are:

1. Glycerine and water
2. Chloroform and benzene.

Procedure

1. 1 ml of blood is collected from syringe; a drop of blood is delivered directly into each of labelled test tubes from a height of about 1 cm from the surface of $CuSO_4$.
2. The drop of blood on entering $CuSO_4$ is surrounded by thin coat of copper proteinate. This layer does not produce any change in density.
3. The drop first falls for 2–3 cm below the surface of solution and loses momentum within a few seconds.
4. If the specific gravity of the drop of blood is greater than $CuSO_4$ then it continues to sink for the next 15–20 sec.
5. If its specific gravity is same as that of the solution, it will remain stationary. If, however, the specific gravity is lower than that of the solution it will raise to the surface.

Precautions

1. The stock solution and standard solution should be carefully prepared.
2. Blood should be dropped from 1 cm above the surface of standard solution. If blood is dropped from a greater height, it will sink to the bottom because of its greater momentum.
3. The reading should be taken 15 to 20 sec. after adding the drop of blood to $CuSO_4$ solution.

Discussion

The normal range of specific gravity of venous blood is 1.005 to 1.065; serum 1.028 to 1.032; corpuscles 1.092 to 1.095. The specific gravity is subjected to physiological and pathological variations.

Physiological

1. It is highest in newborn babies due to polycythemia
2. It is lower in women than men because of comparatively lower RBC count of women.
3. *Pregnancy:* It is lower during pregnancy because of haemodilution due to increase in plasma volume.
4. *Diurnal variation:* It is lower in afternoon and after meals and is higher during night.
5. *Exercise:* It is higher after strenuous exercise due to raised RBC count.
6. *Haemoconcentration:* Less water intake or excessive sweating raises the specific gravity of blood.

Pathological

In conditions like vomiting, diarrhoea and burns, the specific gravity of blood is raised due to haemoconcentration.

Student's Notes

Result

The specific gravity of the sample of blood is..........

QUESTIONS

1. What are the physiological conditions which affect the specific gravity of blood?
2. What are the uses of determining the specific gravity of blood?
3. What happens when blood reacts with $CuSO_4$?
4. In what pathological conditions is specific gravity increased and decreased?
5. What is the specific gravity of:
   a. Plasma
   b. Red cells
   c. Whole blood
6. Define specific gravity.
7. What is the significance of determining the specific gravity of blood?

Student's Notes

Clinical Physiology

Experiment 1: General Examination

Aim

All systemic examinations should be preceded by general examination, to get a general idea about the physical condition of the subject/patient. The student can refer the following books for detailed information regarding physical examination.

1. Hutchison's clinical methods—Hunter and Bomford, published by ELBS and Churchill Livingstone (1985).
2. Physical diagnosis—Vakil and Golwalla, published by MPP Bombay (1986).
3. Clinical examination—John McLeod, published by ELBS.

A properly elicited history followed by a general examination of the patient will clinch on the system which is mainly affected.

The general examination findings which have bearing on a particular system should be given more importance and should not be missed during general examination.

Before starting with general examination, the personal details of the subject should be recorded, i.e. name, age, sex, occupation and address.

1. *Build and nourishment:* Normal person is well built and well nourished. Variations noted may be—moderately built–poorly built. Noting whether person is over weight or under weight can assess nourishment.
2. *Height and weight:* As per Indian standard, the average height of an adult male is about 170 cm and adult female about 160 cm, weight of adult male ranges between 55–75 kg and of female between 45–65 kg.
3. *Pallor:* Is the paleness that appears in skin and mucous membrane due to decrease in haemoglobin content. Examine the lower palpebral conjunctiva for verification of anaemia. Anaemia can occur due to decreased production of RBCs, increased destruction of RBCs, or blood loss.
4. *Icterus:* It is the yellowish discoloration of sclera, mucous membrane and skin due to increase in serum bilirubin above normal—usually above 2 mg%. Verification can be done on the upper sclera. For this elevate the upper eyelid and ask the subject to look down. Bilirubin specifically stains elastic fibers and sclera has got plenty of elastic fibers. Jaundice can develop due to pre-hepatic (haemolytic), hepatic (hepatocellular) and posthepatic (obstructive) causes.
5. *Cyanosis:* Cyanosis is bluish discoloration of skin and mucous membranes, due to increase in concentration of reduced haemoglobin above 5 gm% in capillary blood. Cyanosis can be central or peripheral. Central cyanosis is due to the defective oxygenation in the lungs or due to arterio-venous shunt in the heart. Peripheral cyanosis is due to the stagnation of blood in the periphery. Central cyanosis is verified on the tongue, lips and peripheral on fingertips, ear lobes, tip of nose, etc. Central cyanosis causes—respiratory diseases, congenital cyanotic heart disease. Peripheral cyanosis causes—congestive cardiac failure, inferior vena caval obstruction (cyanosis of lower extremities).
6. *Clubbing:* Clubbing is hyperplasia of soft tissue, in fingers and toes with obliteration of angle between the root of the nail and skin. The tips of fingers and toes appear like "club". This is seen in chronic hypoxia, lung cancer, cirrhosis of liver, ulcerative colitis and subacute bacterial endocarditis.
7. *Lymphadenopathy:* The lymph nodes in the drainage area of any organ are prone to be affected in diseases of that organ. There may be enlargement or tenderness or both. The usual groups of lymph nodes examined are as follows: Cervical group—vertical chain, axillary group—apical, anterior and posterior, para-aortic group, inguinal group, popliteal group and epitrochlear gland.
8. *Oedema:* Oedema is collection of excess fluid in the extracellular spaces, seen in diseases of cardio-

Student's Notes

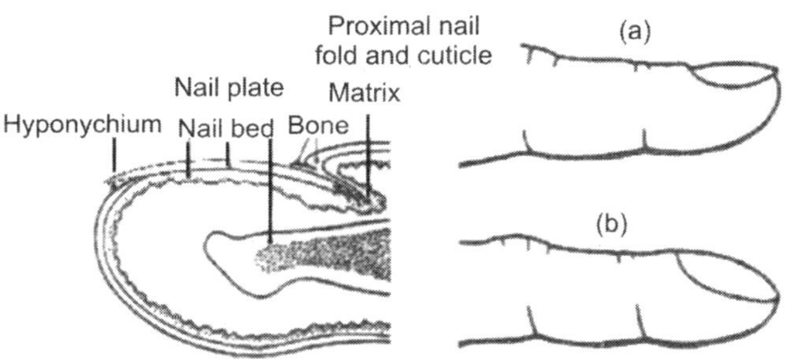

Fig. 1.1: Anatomy of nail: (a) Normal, (b) Clubbing

vascular system, renal system and gastrointestinal system. The mechanism of production varies. Oedema is noted by pressing the area for a sustained period as oedema pits on pressure. In an ambulant patient, oedema develops over lower extremities. In a recumbent patient, oedema develops over the sacral region and back.

9. *Skin and hair:* The colour and texture of skin and abnormalities, if any, should be noted. Similarly the colour and distribution of hair also should be noted.
10. *Pulse:* By definition, it is the expansile impulse transmitted along the arteries, due to the intermittent ejection of blood from the aorta. The features of the pulse to be noted are:
    - Rate—how many per minute.
    - Rhythm—the regularity with which one pulse follows the other.
    - Volume—the amplitude of expansion of vessel wall.
    - Character—whether collapsing or not (rise, maintenance and fall); the contour of a pulse.
    - Condition of vessels wall—thickened or not.
    - Other peripheral pulsations, i.e. brachial, carotid, facial, femoral, popliteal, dorsalis pedis and posterior tibial.
    - Radiofemoral delay—whether there is any time lapse between the appearance of radial and femoral pulsations noted only in CVS diseases.
11. *Blood pressure:* The BP is noted in recumbent and erect postures on the upper limb.
12. *Jugular venous pressure (JVP):* The right internal jugular vein is taken for the study. Keep the subject in a propped up position at 45° inclination to the bed and note the upper level of jugular pulse. The vertical height from sternal angle to the upper level of pulse is taken in centimeters and is expressed as the jugular venous pressure. Normally, the jugular venous pulse is not visible above the clavicle.
13. *Respiratory rate:* Place the right palm over the upper part of the abdomen of the subject and count the number of respirations in one minute.

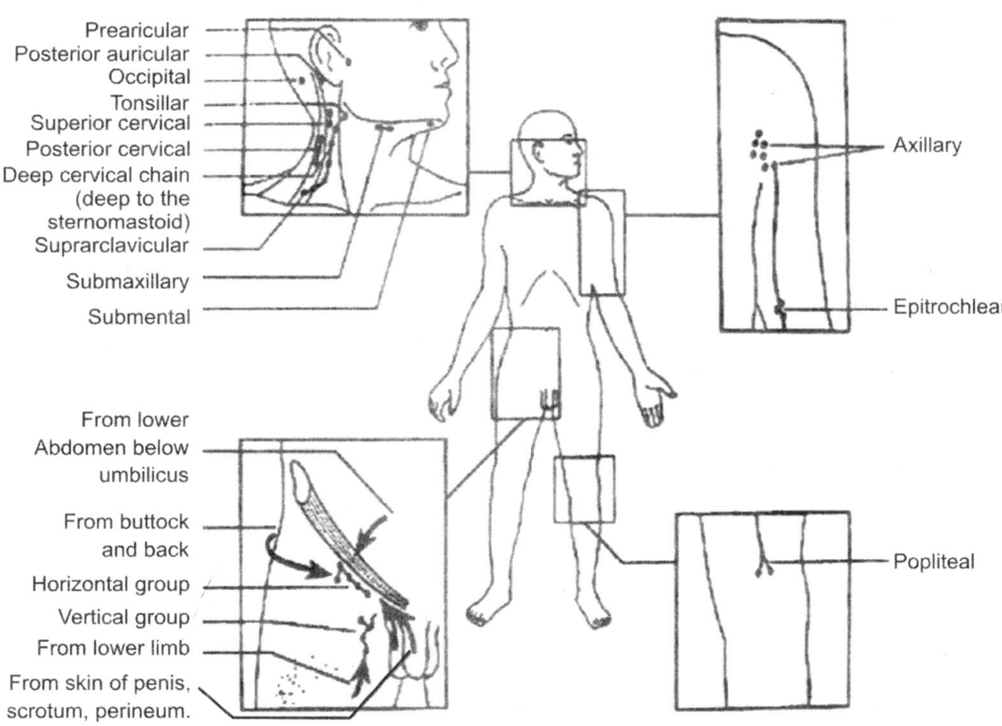

Fig. 1.2: Distribution of palpable lymph glands

Student's Notes

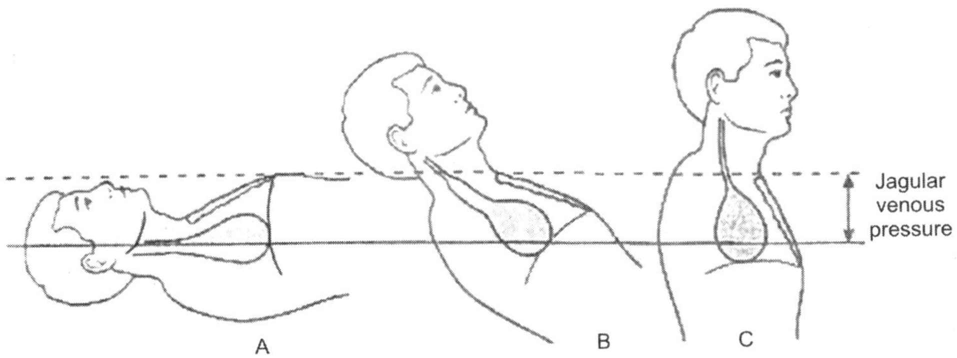

Fig. 1.3: Understanding jugular venous pressure

14. *Body temperature:* Body temperature is measured using the clinical thermometer. Usually, the oral temperature is measured. The subject is asked to hold the thermometer under the tongue, gently supported by the lips for two minutes. The procedure should not be done immediately after taking hot or cold drinks. In unconscious patients, rectal temperature is usually taken and in young children, either axillary temperature or rectal temperature can be taken.

In addition to above-mentioned points, the following should be specially noted, if relevant.

Along with cardiovascular and respiratory system:
- Dyspnoea
- Cough
- Chest pain
- Sputum

Along with central nervous system:
- Neurofibromas
- Tuft of hair on low back
- Short neck
- Pes cavus, pes planus
- Polydactyly, syndactyly
- Haemangiomas

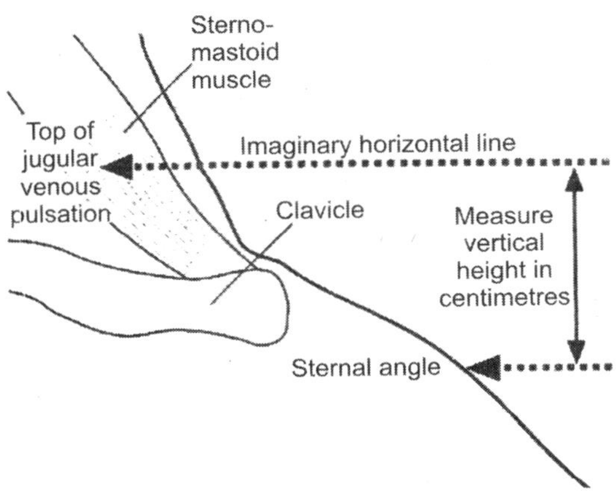

Fig. 1.4: Measuring jugular venous pressure

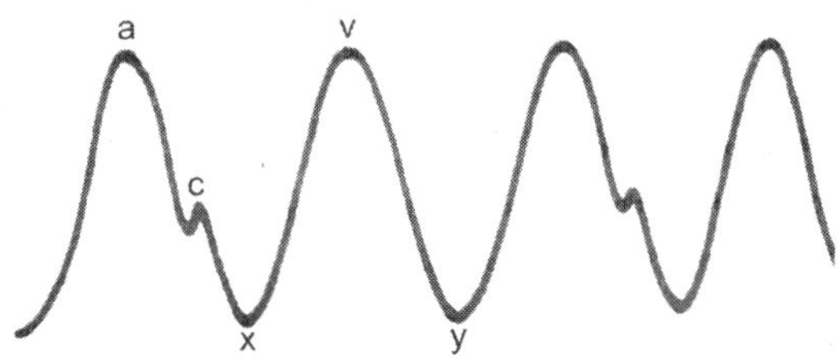

Fig. 1.5: The normal venous pulse

REPORT

Name :
Age :
Occupation :
Address :

General Examination

Well built and well nourished
Height 170 cm
Weight 60 kg

No pallor, no icterus, no cyanosis
No clubbing of fingers or toes
No significant lymph node enlargement
No oedema
Skin, hair and nails appear healthy.

Pulse: 72/min regular, normal in volume and character, no thickening of vessel walls, all peripheral pulsations are felt equally on both sides and there is no radio-femoral delay.

Blood pressure: 120/80 mm Hg in the right upper limb in supine position.

JVP : Not raised
Respiratory rate : 18/min, regular
Body temperature : 37°C

Impression: On general examination, the subject appears to be normal.

Student's Notes

Experiment 2: Examination of the Respiratory System

Aim

To perform the clinical examination of the respiratory system on a given subject. Examination of the respiratory system is done on the following headings:

1. Inspection
2. Palpation
3. Percussion
4. Auscultation

INSPECTION

The subject is stripped up to the waist and is examined under good light. The following points are noted:

1. Position of the trachea and the apex beat
2. Shape of the chest and deformities
3. Respiratory rate
4. Type of breathing
5. Movements of the chest
6. Any wasting of muscles or drooping of the shoulder.

The shape of the chest is normally bilaterally symmetrical and varies with the build of the individual. It is short, broad and deep in thick fat individuals: long, narrow, and flat in thin tall people. It is barrel-shaped in emphysematous condition. The cross-section of the chest in a normal person is some what elliptical. Ratio between anteroposterior and transverse diameters being 5:7. The rate, rhythm, type of respiration and chest movement during respiration are noted. It is regular in rhythm and abdominothoracic in adults and in young children and in women it is thoraco-abdominal during pregnancy. The expansion of the chest is equal on both sides.

PALPATION

Mediastinal position: The position of the trachea is determined by placing the index finger and the ring finger on the bony prominences of the suprasternal notch and the middle finger is gently pushed posteriorly and downwards between the sterno-cleidomastoid and the trachea on either side to see for any tracheal deviation.

The position of the apex beat is also palpated. Displacement of trachea and/or apex beat may occur in mediastinal shift due to disease of the lungs or pleura.

Chest movement: To determine the chest expansion of the apical region of the lungs, the hands are placed over the shoulders close to the neck and the thumb at right angle to other fingers and approximated in the midline (This is carried out with the examiner standing behind the subject).

To determine the expansion of the other regions, the chest is gripped on either side and thumbs approximated in the midline. When the subject takes full inspiration, the distance of departure of the thumbs from the midline indicates the extent of expansion of either half of the chest.

Vocal fremitus: These are vibrations that are felt on the chest wall when the subject utters a sound. To test vocal fremitus, the subject is told to repeat "one, one". The palm or ulnar border of the hand is applied flat on the chest. The intensity of vibration is compared on corresponding areas of the two sides of the chest. Vocal fremitus is increased in consolidation of lung and diminished in pleural effusion.

Expansion of the chest: The degree of expansion of chest may be measured by placing an inch tape just below the nipple around the chest with its mark at the middle of the sternum. Instruct the subject to breathe in and out as deep as possible. In females, the mammary tissue is avoided by making the measurement above or below the mammary gland. Initial respiratory efforts are often shallow. So readings are taken after 2 or 3 breaths. Measure the chest circumference at the end of deep inspiration and at the end of deep expiration 5 to 8 cm difference is normal. It is decreased in bronchial asthma, pulmonary fibrosis, etc.

PERCUSSION

There are two types of percussion:

i. Direct and
ii. Indirect

In direct percussion, the clavicle is percussed directly. In indirect percussion, the middle finger of the left hand (pleximeter finger) is placed firmly parallel to the inter costal space. The back of the middle phalanx is struck perpendicularly with the tip of the middle finger of the right hand (percussing finger). Rules to be followed during percussion are:

1. The stroke should be delivered at the wrist and finger joint, not at the elbow or shoulder.
2. The long axis of the pleximeter finger should be parallel to the edge of the organ being percussed.
3. Percussion should be done from a resonant area to a dull area.

Student's Notes

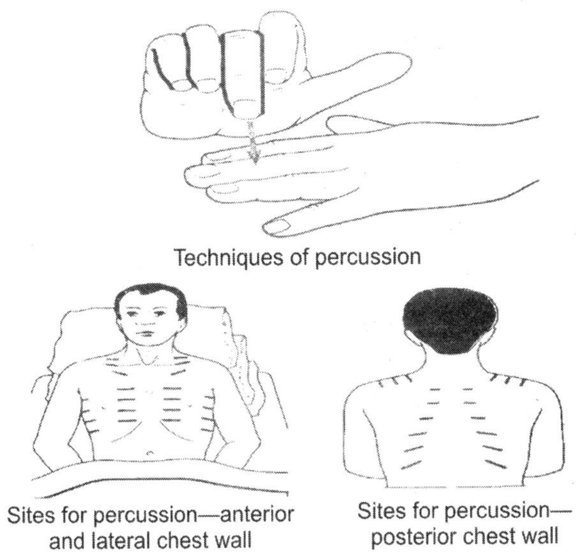

Fig. 2.1: Techniques of percussion

During percussion of the sides of the chest, the subject's hands are placed over the head and while percussing the back of the chest, the subject is asked to criss-cross his arms in front of him. Lung resonance is impaired in consolidations and fibrosis. In thickened pleura and pleural effusion, stony dullness occurs. Resonance is increased in pneumothorax.

AUSCULTATION

Auscultation is performed all over the chest. Corresponding points on either side is to be auscultated simultaneously. The character of breath sounds, vocal resonance and abnormal sounds if any are noted.

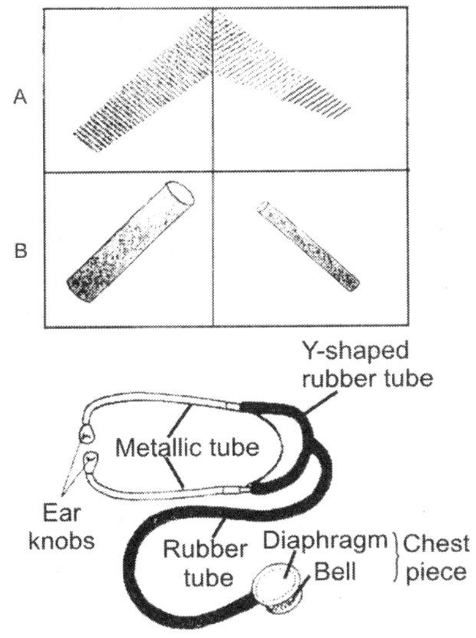

Fig. 2.2: Stethoscope (Littman's type)

1. Character of Breath Sounds

There are two typical varieties of breath sounds: (a) vesicular and (b) bronchial.

Vesicular breath sounds: These are heard all over the chest under normal conditions. The inspiratory sounds are intense and audible during the whole of inspiration. Expiratory sound follows that of inspiration without a distinct pause, and is audible only during the early part of expiration. Vesicular breath sounds are low pitched and rustling in character.

Bronchial breath sounds: These are produced by the passage of air through the trachea and large bronchi. The inspiratory sound is moderately intense, becomes inaudible before the end of inspiration. The duration extends through the greater part of expiration, being as long as the inspiratory sound.

Tubular breath sound: High pitched bronchial breath sound heard over the consolidated lung tissue.

Cavernous breath sound: Low pitched bronchial breathing heard over large cavities. Diminution or absence of breath sounds are found when there is thickened pleura, pleural effusion and pneumothorax. It will also be found in condition causing diminished air entry to the underlying lung.

2. Vocal Resonance

These are auscultatory sounds when the subject is repeatedly saying 'one, one, one' vocal resonance is increased in consolidation, diminished in pleural thickening, pleural effusion and pneumothorax.

3. Abnormal Sounds

These are rhonchi, crepitations and pleural rub, which are heard during diseased condition of the lung.

Rhonchi are heard when there is narrowing of the respiratory passage and crepitations or rales are heard when there is presence of fluid secretions. Rub is grating sounds heard during pleurisy.

Observation

Respiratory system examination of the given subject is found to be normal.

QUESTIONS

1. What is sternal angle?
2. What is the normal position of trachea? Why?
3. What is the difference between vocal resonance and vocal fremitus?
4. What are the abnormal shapes of the chest?

Student's Notes

5. What are the rules of percussion?
6. Define the term eupnoea, tachypnoea, apnoea, dyspnoea and hyperpnoea?
7. What is pleural effusion?
8. What are added sounds? When do they occur?
9. What are the causes for a shift in the mediastinum?
10. What is the cause for the slightly increased vocal resonance in the right upper zone of the normal lung?
11. Where are bronchial breath sounds heard in the normal human?
12. Where are vesicular breath sounds heard well in the normal human?
13. What is the significance of noting the positions of the trachea and apex?
14. Fill in the Table

	Percussion	*Breath sounds*	*Vocal resonance*
Pleural effusion	Stony dullness	Decrease	Decrease
Consolidation	Dull	Bronchial sounds even over other parts	Increase
Pneumothorax	Hyper-resonance	Decrease	Decrease

15. Define BBS and VBS and what is the difference?

	Bronchial breath sounds	*Vesicular breath sounds*
Produced by	Large airways	Small airways
Pitch	High pitch & harsh	Low pitch (rustle)
Pause between I & E*	Present	Absent
Relative duration of I & E	Equal	E < I

* I = inspiration E = expiration

16. What are the investigations that can be done in diseases of the respiratory system?

Student's Notes

RESPIRATORY SYSTEM

Name: .... Age:....................

Sex: .... Occupation: ....

General Examination

Build and nutrition ....

Pallor ....

Icterus ....

Cyanosis ....

Arterial pulse ....

BP ....

Temp ....

Clubbing ....

Lymphadenopathy ....

Pedal edema ....

Systemic Examination

Inspection
- Chest and spine shape ....
- Any obvious wasting ....
- Trachea ....
- Apex beat ....
- Type of breathing ....
- Respiratory rate ....
- Chest movements ....
- Chest symmetry ....
- Scars, sinuses ....

Palpation
- Trachea ....
- Apex beat ....
- Chest movements ....
- Chest expansion ....
- Vocal fremitus * on both sides ....

Percussion
- Direct (both sides) ....
- Indirect* ....

Auscultation
- Breath sounds* ....
- Vocal resonance* ....
- Adventitious sounds ....

Report

The respiratory system of the subject was examined in detail and was found to be normal.

- Draw a table as given below for the points marked by star.

	Right	Left
1. Supraclavicular		
2. Infraclavicular		
3. Mammary		
4. Axillary		
5. Infra-axillary		
6. Supra-scapular		
7. Inter-scapular		
Upper		
Middle		
Lower		
8. Infra-scapular		

Student's Notes

Experiment 3: Recording of Respiratory Movements (Stethography)

Aim

To record the movements of respiration.

Principle

It consists of a corrugated rubber tube with a stopper at each end and air outlet pipe connected to the tambour. If a rubber tube is tied round the chest, the movement of thorax during respiration brings about a change in the pressure of air contained in tube. This change in pressure of air inside the rubber tube can be recorded by connecting the tube to a suitable recording device.

Requirements

1. Sherrington-Starling's drum (S.S. drum)
2. Stethograph
3. Marey's tambour.

Procedure

The subject is allowed to sit on a stool. The stethograph which is connected to a Marey's tambour is tied around the chest of the subject. The S.S. drum is allowed to move at 1.2 mm/sec speed and the writing point of piston recorder is brought into contact with the smoked paper on the drum. First the normal respiratory movements are recorded. The subject is asked, to take forceful, deep and rapid respirations for 3 seconds and the record is continued till normal movement return. The subject is asked to swallow a glass of water and its effect on respiratory movements are recorded. The subject is asked to breathe in and out into a polythene bag and a record of the effect of CO_2 excess is obtained. The subject is asked to take maximum forceful inspiration and to hold his breathe for as long as he can. The movement of the chest during breath holding and the return to normal respiration is recorded. The effect of exercise on respiration are also recorded (effects of other manoeuvres may also be recorded). A time tracing is taken by an electrical time marker (frequency 1/sec) below the record of respiratory movements and the normal respiration rate is calculated. The tracings after being labelled are fixed in the varnishing fluid.

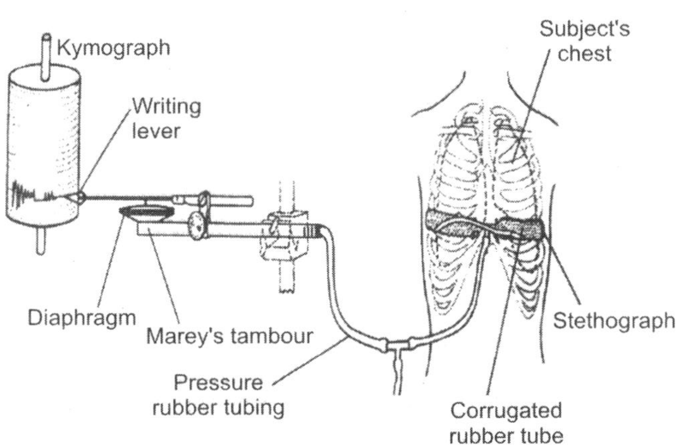

Fig. 3.1: Stethograph

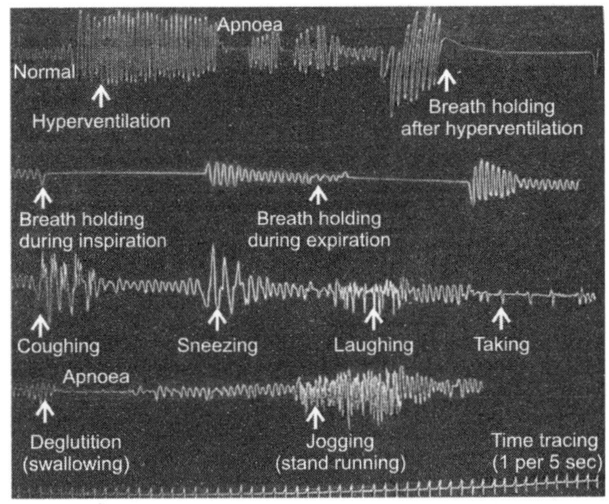

Fig. 3.2: Stethograph recording

QUESTIONS

1. What changes occur following hyperventilation, swallowing and apnoea?
2. Outline the mechanism by which arterial blood pCO_2, affects respiration?
3. What are the effects of exercise on respiration?
4. How else may respiration be recorded?
5. What is the mechanism of the apnoea or hypoventilation, which follows voluntary hyperventilation?
6. What is periodic breathing? Mention the conditions where this develops. What is its mechanism?
7. What is the cause of the hyperventilation following breath holding?
8. Define apnoea. Classify apnoea?
9. What are the uses of stethography?
10. What is the principle involved in stethography?
11. What is the normal breath-holding time in adults?
12. What is breaking point?

Student's Notes

STETHOGRAPHY

Name : .... Age: ....

Sex: .... Occupation: ....

Manoeuver	*Effect seen*
1. Normal breathing	
2. Hyperventilation	
3. Breath holding	
4. Deglutition	
5. Coughing	
6. Sneezing	
7. Laughing	
8. Talking	
9. Jogging	

Inference:

Student's Notes

Experiment 4: Spirometry

Aim

To record and measure vital capacity, tidal volume and expiratory reserve volume in a given subject.

Several models of spirometers are available out of which student's spirometer is very commonly used in the laboratory. It consists of a metal cylinder of adequate capacity, which is filled with water. A metal tube pierces the bottom of the cylinder and rises above the level of the water. This metallic tube at one end is connected by a rubber tubing with mouthpiece, into which the subject breathes. The spirometer bell is another metallic cylinder of slightly smaller diameter. It is completely submerged in the water and its weight is balanced by a counter weight. The top of the spirometer bell is connected by a cord running over a pulley to a weight. The subject's nose is clipped and through the mouthpiece breathes out into the spirometer and the air raises the bell. The volume of air is read from the scale marked on the pulley. The inner cylinder is raised initially and the subject may be asked to breathe in from it to measure inspiratory volumes.

Procedure

1. Sterilize the mouthpiece with spirit.
2. Adjust the pointer on the pulley to the zero mark with the drum pushed down and confirm that the pointer moves in the correct direction on pulling the drum up.

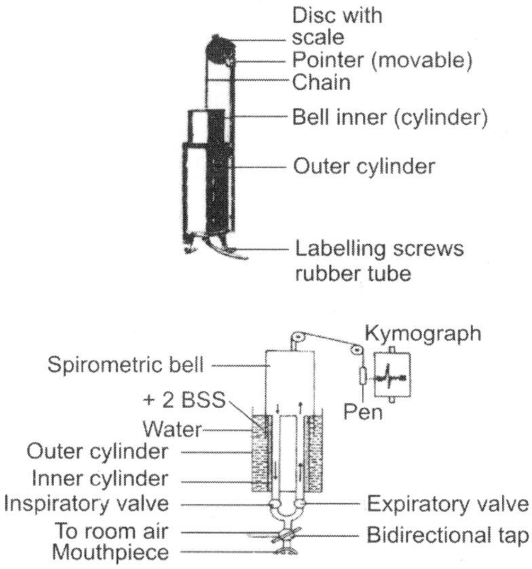

Fig. 4.1: Spirometer

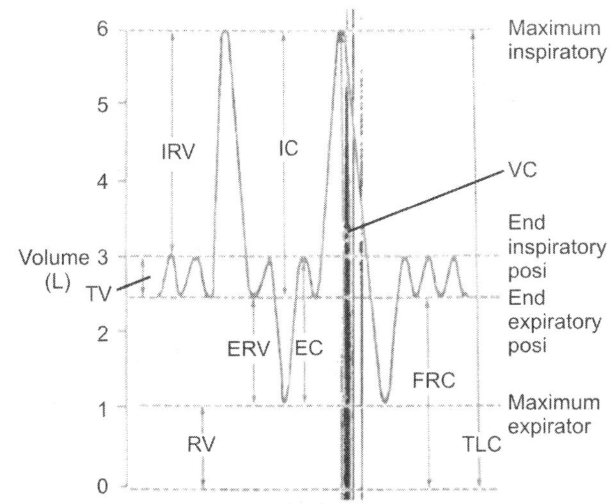

Fig. 4.2: Aspirogram

3. Breathe at tidal volume, at the end of normal inspiration breathe out as usual but into the mouthpiece. The volume recorded is the tidal volume.
4. Readjust the drum at the lower position with pointer at zero. Breathe again at tidal volume. At the end of normal expiration, breathe out forcibly into the mouthpiece till you can breathe out no more. This volume is the expiratory reserve volume.
5. Readjust the spirometer as in step 4. After a few tidal breaths, breathe in maximally and breathe out maximally into the mouthpiece. This reading is the vital capacity.

QUESTIONS

1. Define tidal volume, vital capacity, IRV, ERV, maximum breathing capacity (MBC).
2. What are the factors, which will affect the vital capacity?
3. What is functional residual capacity and residual volume (FRC and RV)?
4. How would you measure FRC and RV?
5. What is respiratory reserve?
6. What is dyspnoeic index?
7. Draw a schematic diagram of a spirometer.
8. What is the effect of change in posture on vital capacity? Explain.
9. Give its normal values of vital capacity in an adult male and female.

SPIROMETRY

Name: ....
Age: ....

Occupation: ....
Sex: ....

Lung volume capacity	*Reading 1*	*Reading 2*	*Reading 3*
Vital capacity Inspiratory reserve volume Expiratory reserve volume Tidal volume			

Inference:

Student's Notes

Experiment 5: Respiratory Efficiency Tests

Aim

To determine the efficiency of respiratory system.

Requirements

1. Sphygmomanometer
2. Stopwatch
3. Mini-peak flow meter

Procedure

a. *Breath holding test:* Ask the subject to breath out as deeply as possible and to take in air as much as possible. Now, ask him to hold his breath to the breaking point and determine the maximum time with a stop watch, noting the subjective symptoms during the experiment.

b. *40 mm endurance test:* After a deep expiration, ask the subject to inspire to the maximum. Now apply a clip to the nose and ask him to expire into the mercury manometer up to the level 40 mm and to maintain it as long as possible. Record the maximum possible

c. *Peak expiratory flow rate (PEFR):* After a deep inspiration, ask the subject to expire forcefully into the mouthpiece of the mini-peak flow meter after adjusting the knob to the zero level.

d. *Candle test or expiratory blast test*

Result

1. Maximum breath holding time =
2. Maximum endurance time =
3. PEFR =

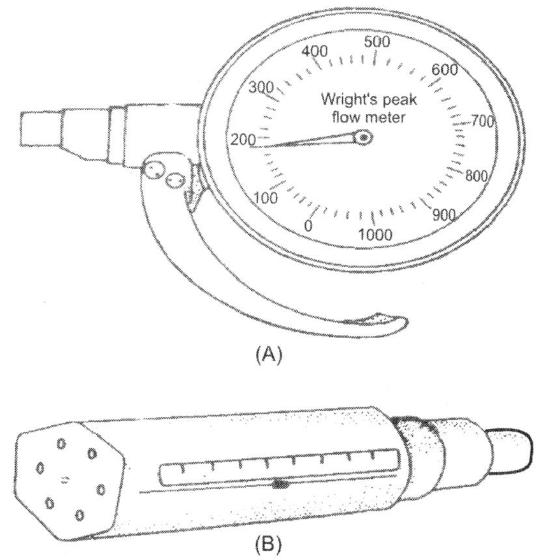

Fig. 5.1: Wright's peak flow meter (A) and mini-right peak flow meter (B)

QUESTIONS

1. What is the standard breath holding time?
2. What is the normal maximal endurance time?
3. What is breaking point?
4. Define PEFR? What is the normal value?
5. Define VC, FEV? How is it useful?
6. Define MVV or MBC?
7. What is Dyspnoeic index?
8. In what situation is respiratory efficiency test assessed?
9. What is expiratory blast test? (Candle test)
10. Does the PEFR and VC correlate well?

RESPIRATORY EFFICIENCY TESTS

Name: .... Occupation: ....

Age: .... Sex: ....

	1	2	3
Maximum breath-holding test			
Maximum endurance test			
PEFR			

Inference:

Student's Notes

Experiment 6: Examination of the Cardiovascular System

Aim

Examination of the cardiovascular system includes examination of the heart as well as the blood vessels. The cardiovascular system is assessed in the following order:

1. Arterial pulses
2. Blood pressure
3. Venous pulses
4. Examination of the precordium (part of the chest which overlies the heart)

Anatomical Landmarks

1. Sternal angle or the angle of Louis. This marks the junction of the manubrium with the body of the sternum. The second costal cartilage articulates with the sternum at this level. The space immediately above this is the first intercostal space.
2. *Midclavicular line:* Vertical line descending from the center of clavicle.
3. Anterior, mid and posterior axillary lines are vertical lines descending respectively from the anterior border, the centre and posterior border of the axilla.

Arterial Pulses

The presence or absence of the main peripheral pulses—the radial, brachial, carotid, femoral, popliteal, posterior tibial and dorsalis pedis pulses are noted. The volume of each was compared with the other side.

Method of Examining the Pulse

The pulse is usually felt at the wrist and over the radial artery because of its superficial position. It is best felt with the subject's forearm slightly pronated and the wrist flexed. The examiner's three finger, viz. the index, middle and ring finger should be over the radial artery. Both radial arteries are palpated simultaneously to detect the irregularities of the pulse on the two sides. The following observations are to be made with regard to cardiac function.

1. *Rate of pulse:* It is stated as so many beats per minute. The normal pulse rate is about 70 to 80 per minute (to be precise 60–100 beats is considered normal). Increase in pulse rate (tachycardia) occurs during fever and in thyrotoxicosis. Decrease in pulse rate (bradycardia) occurs in myxoedema and following regular athletic training. Abnormalities of the function of SA or AV nodes may reduce the heart rate. Pulse deficit: The difference between the heart rate and the pulse rate is called as pulse deficit.

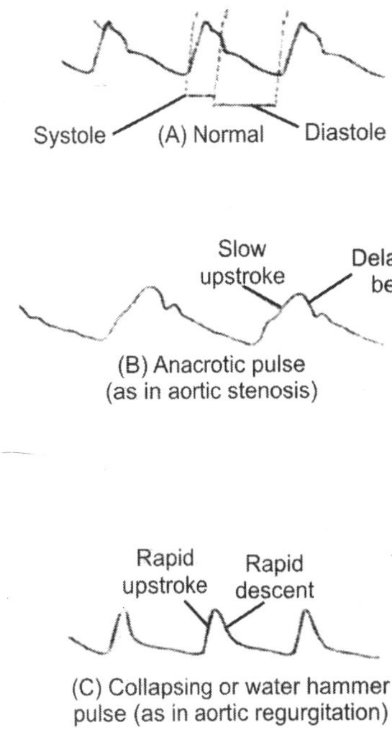

Fig. 6.1

2. *Rhythm:* The rhythm could be regular or irregular. It could be regularly irregular or irregularly irregular Regularly irregular pulse would be seen during atrial extrasystole which occurs at a regular interval. Irregularly irregular pulse would be seen in atrial fibrillation.
3. *Character:* The character or form of the pulse wave is studied by palpating the carotid pulse.
   a. *Collapsing (water-hammer) pulse:* Characterized by a rapid up stroke and descent of the pulse wave. It would be seen in large arteriovenous communications.
   b. *Pulsus paradoxus:* There is a marked diminution in an arterial pressure as seen in pericardial effusion.
   c. Pulsus alternans occur when the left ventricular muscle is severely failing. The ventricle beats strongly and then weakly, in successive beats of normal rhythm.
4. *Volume:* This gives a rough guide to pulse pressure. Which depends upon the stroke volume and the compliance of the arteries. With normal vessels, the pulse volume gives an indication of the stroke volume.

Student's Notes

5. *Nature of the vessel wall:* Vessel wall is thickened in old age due to atherosclerosis.
6. *Radiofemoral delay:* Delay of the femoral pulse compared with the rt. radial pulse is found in coarctation of the aorta.

Blood Pressure

It is to be measured by the following methods.

1. Palpatory
2. Auscultatory
3. Oscillatory

Venous Pulses

Examination of the neck veins especially the internal jugular vein is done with the patient in a good light and inclined at an angle of about 45°. The neck is supported so that the neck muscles, especially the sternomastoid are relaxed. The normal slight pulsations of the veins and the three waves (a, c and v waves) are distinguished.

There is a mean level and the perpendicular height of this level above the right atrium indicates the mean hydrostatic pressure within the right atrium. The normal upper limit is 4 cm vertically above, the sternal angle . This is about 9 cm above the right atrium. In a healthy person reclining at an angle of 45° the mean level will be invisible because it is just below the clavicle

Elevation of the JVP indicates elevation of the right atrial pressure.

Causes of Elevation of JVP

1. Congestive heart failure
2. Pulmonary embolism
3. Constrictive pericarditis
4. Tricuspid valve disease.

Arterial pulsation may also be visible in the neck and has to be distinguished from various pulsations.

1. Venous pulse has a definite upper level.
2. This level falls during inspiration.
3. Firm but gentle pressure on the upper abdomen will raise the level due to transient increase in the venous return. (hepatojugular reflux).
4. Venous pulsation is not palpable.
5. It is more sinuous and less sharp than arterial pulsation.

The venous pulsations are more easily recognised in external jugular veins than in internal jugular veins but the former is less reliable because:

1. Of the presence of venous valves within the external jugular system.
2. It passes through more fascial planes so that it is more likely to be affected by external compression.

Examination of the Precordium

The precordium is to be examined in the following order:

- Inspection
- Palpation
- Percussion
- Auscultation

Inspection: The subject is stripped up to the waist and the chest wall is examined for any deformities. Some of the common deformities include pigeon chest, barrel chest (cylindrical chest), funnel-shaped chest (exaggeration of the normal hollow over the lower end of sternum).

The position of trachea is noted. The position and the extent of the apical impulse are made out. The apical impulse is the lower most and the outer most point of definite cardiac pulsation. The normal position of the apical beat is 1 cm internal to the mid-clavicular line in the left fifth intercostal space.

Any other pulsations or engorged veins over the chest wall or the presence of extrathoracic, pulse are also noted for.

Palpation: The position of trachea is confirmed. This method confirms the inspection findings. The apical impulse is to be felt initially with the palmar aspect of the hand and finally localised by the digital method. Abnormal impulse, if any like 'thrill' is to be made out by palpation. 'Thrill' is palpable murmur.

The apex beat may be displaced due to disease of the surrounding viscera which 'push' or 'pull' from the usual site.

Causes of 'pushing' are:

1. Pleural effusion
2. Pneumothorax

Causes of 'pulling' are:

1. Pulmonary fibrosis
2. Collapse of lung

Enlargement of the heart can also cause displacement of the apex beat outwards.

Percussion: The left border of the heart is percussed first and then the right border.

Left border of the heart: The apex beat is to be marked by percussing from a resonant area in the axilla and moving inside at the fifth intercostal space. Like wise the left border is to be marked by percussing intercostal space above, moving from axilla inwards.

Right border of the heart: Percussion is to be done from above downwards in the intercostal spaces on the right side till the liver dullness is reached. Then percussion in the intercostal space just above the liver dullness is

Student's Notes

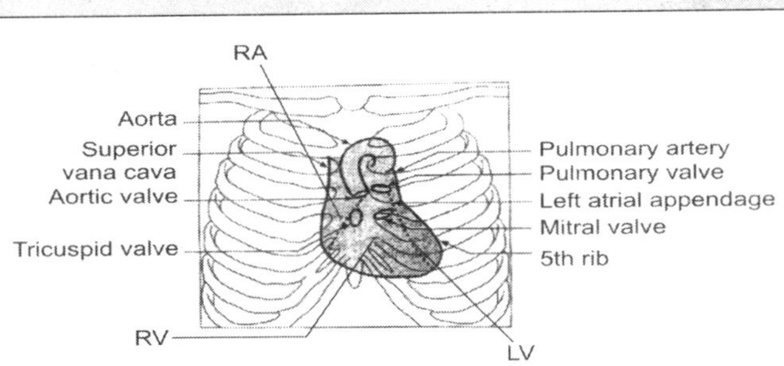

Fig. 6.2

made from outside inwards to mark the lower boundary of the organ. Similar percussion is to be made on the intercostals space at a higher level, from outside inwards to mark the right border.

Joining the lower limit of the left and right borders and the upper limit of the same gives the inferior and superior borders of the heart. Superior border may be percussed for starting at the topmost intercostal space on the left side.

Auscultations: Auscultation is done by means of a stethoscope. The important auscultatory areas are:

1. Mitral area. Corresponds to the apex beat.
2. Tricuspid area. lies just to the left of the lower end of sternum.
3. Aortic area. lies to the right of the sternum in the second intercostal space.
4. Pulmonary area. lies to the left of the sternum in the second intercostal space.

These areas are customarily called by the name of the valve from which murmurs and sounds arise. This does not correspond to the anatomical location of the valves.

Heart Sounds

Clinically two heart sounds are easily distinguishable. The first heart sound is due to the closure of the AV valves (mitral and tricuspid), usually pronounced as 'Lub'. It synchronises with the carotid pulse beat.

The second heart sound is due to the closure of the semilunar valves (aortic and pulmonary), usually pronounced as 'Dub'.

In disease, the following deviations from the normal occur.

1. The sounds may have different intensity, either increased or decreased.
2. The sounds may be abnormally split.
3. Low frequency sounds in diastole—third and fourth heart sounds may be heard.
4. Additional sounds, often related to abnormal valves may be heard.

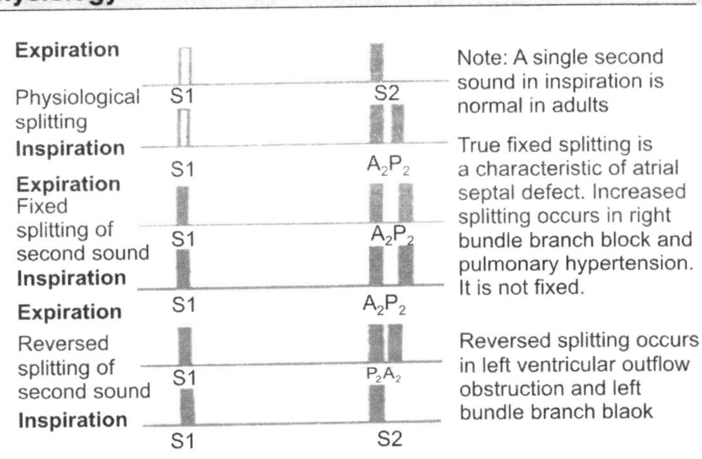

Fig. 6.3

Observation

The cardiovascular system of the given subject is normal.

QUESTIONS

1. What is precordium?
2. How will you identify the intercostal space?
3. What is the normal shape of the chest?
4. What is orthopnoea and paroxysmal nocturnal dyspnoea?
5. Name the four auscultatory areas—their exact positions?
6. What is apical impulse? What is the normal site?
7. Why JVP is seen on the right side of the neck? What is their normal level?
8. When dose JVP get increased? Name the jugular venous waves after drawing it.
9. What are the abnormal pulses you know?
10. Why is radial artery always chosen? What information can you get on palpating the artery?
11. When does the vessel wall get thickened?
12. What are the types of irregular pulse you know?
13. What is a murmur?
14. Clinically how will you identify the 1st heart sound?
15. When is 1st heart sound loud?
16. When is 2nd heart sound loud?
17. What is the cause of 3rd HS and 4th HS? What is its significance?
18. When do you get a
    - Systolic murmur
    - Diastolic murmur
    - Continuous murmur
19. What is phonocardiogram and echocardiogram?

Student's Notes

20. What is the physiological basis for the "split" of the 2nd heart sound?
21. What are the heart sounds other than those mentioned above caused by?
22. Which portion of the heart corresponds to the
    a. Apex
    b. Parasternal area
23. What is a "Bruit"?
24. Enter the timing of the murmurs in the table provided.

Valve	*Lesion*	*Timing*
Aortic	Stenosis	Systole (ventricular)
Pulmonary	Regurgitation	Diastole (ventricular)
Mitral	Stenosis	Diastole (ventricular)
Tricuspid	Regurgitation	Systole (ventricular)

25. What other positions would you like to put the patient to feel the apical impulse?

CARDIOVASCULAR SYSTEM OBSERVATION

Name: .... Age: ....

Sex: .... Occupation: ....

General Examination

Build and nutritional status ....

Pallor ....

Icterus ....

Cyanosis ....

Clubbing ....

Lymphadenopathy ....

Pedal edema ....

Arterial pulse: Rate, rhythm, volume, character, condition of vessel wall, radio femoral delay, pulse-apex deficit, all peripheral pulses.

BP ....

Temp ....

JVP ....

Systemic examination ....

Inspection
- Trachea ....
- Apex-beat ....
- Venous engorgement............................
- Chest and spine shape ....
- Scars ....

Palpation
- Trachea ....
- Apex beat ....
- Thrills ....

Percussion
- Right border ....
- Left border ....
- Superior border ....

Auscultation
- Mitral area ....
- Tricuspid area S1, S2 murmurs ....
- Pulmonary area other sounds ....
- Aortic area ....

Report

The cardiovascular system of the given subject was examined in detail and was found to be normal.

Student's Notes

Experiment 7: Determination of the Blood Pressure

Definition

Blood pressure is the lateral pressure exerted by the column of blood on the wall of the artery.

Aim

To determine the blood pressure of subject at rest and after moderate exercise.

Apparatus

Sphygmomanometer, stethoscope.

Principle

The pressure of blood in the artery (brachial artery) is balanced against the pressure of air in a rubber cuff surrounding the artery. The pressure of air in the cuff is then measured by means of a mercury manometer.

Methods

1. Palpatory method.
2. Auscultatory method.
3. Oscillatory method.

Procedure

1. *Palpatory method:* The subject is asked to sit on a stool. The cuff is tied around the upper arm with the lower border of the cuff not less than 2.5 cm, above the cubital fossa. The outlet valve of the bulb is closed. The radial pulse is palpated while the cuff is being inflated to a pressure slightly above the level at which the radial pulsation is no longer felt. The pressure at which the pulsation was obliterated is read in the mercury manometer. The outlet valve is opened. The manometric reading is noted at the point where the pulsation reappeared. The average of the two readings gives the systolic pressure. The diastolic pressure cannot be determined by this method.
2. *Auscultatory method:* By palpatory method, only the systolic blood pressure could be measured. By auscultatory method, both the systolic and diastolic blood pressure can be measured.
   The chest piece of the stethoscope is placed over the brachial artery. The pressure in the cuff is raised above the systolic pressure (by about 30 mmHg) previously determined by the palpatory method. The pressure is then lowered gradually (2–3 mm per second). The sounds that are heard are the Korotkoff's sounds. The first sound (phase one) that occurs is a sharp tapping sound, indicates the peak systolic pressure, the second and third phases initially murmurish in quality and then louder and more banging, are due to turbulent flow of blood through a partially occluded vessel. In the fourth phase, the sound becomes muffled and dull and the fifth phase accurately gives true diastolic pressure, which is disappearance of the sound.
3. *Oscillatory method:* This is another method of determining blood pressure. By this method, both the systolic and diastolic blood pressure are determined. The pressure at which oscillations appear in the mercury manometer gives the systolic pressure and the pressure at which it disappears gives the diastolic blood pressure. However, this method is not accurate.

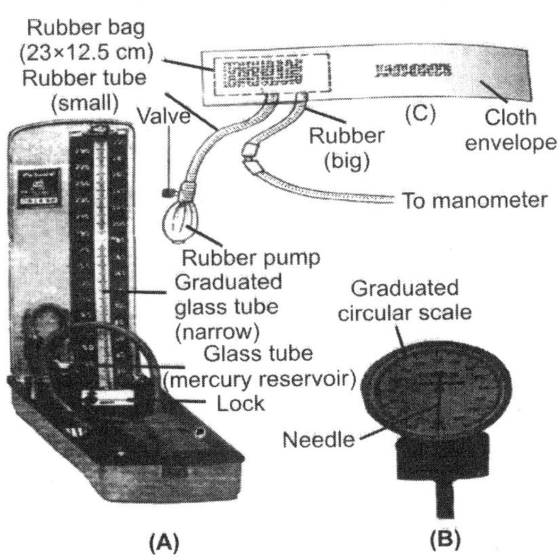

Fig. 7.1: Sphygmomanometer

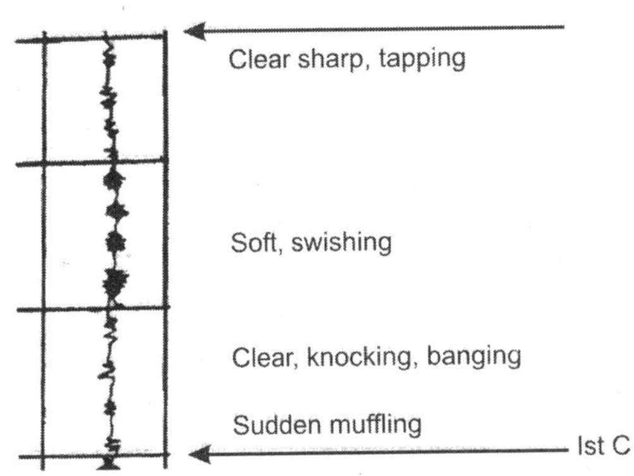

Fig. 7.2

Student's Notes

Important Precautions in the uses of Sphygmomanometer

1. The manometer should be placed at the level of the heart.
2. The lower border of the *cuff* should be 2.5 cm above the cubital fossa. For children, a narrow cuff should be used.
3. Blood pressure should be preferably taken in the left arm.

Normal Values

The average systolic pressure in healthy adults is 100–140 mm Hg. The average diastolic pressure is 60–90 mm Hg. In children, it is closer to the lower end of the scale and in the elderly it reaches or even exceeds the higher figure. The difference between the systolic and diastolic pressure is the pulse pressure 30–60 mm Hg.

Other Physiological Variations

Blood pressure is slightly lower in women than men. Persons with slender build have got a lower blood pressure that those of heavy build. During sleep, systolic pressure is less. Emotional excitement and muscular exercise cause an increase in the blood pressure. It is also increased after meals. The blood pressure especially the diastolic is highest in the standing position, lower in the sitting and lowest while the subject is lying down.

Pathological Increase in Blood Pressure

1. Essential hypertension
2. Adrenal tumour
3. Hyperthyroidism
4. Pheochromocytoma.

Pathological Decrease in Blood Pressure

1. In shock
2. Hypothyroidism
3. In adrenal insufficiency.

Discussion

Blood pressure is the lateral pressure exerted by the column of blood on the wall of the vessels while flowing through it.

Systolic pressure is the maximum pressure in the arteries during systole. It indicates:

a. The extent of work done by the heart.
b. The force with which the heart is working
c. The degree of pressure which the arterial walls have to withstand. Normal systolic pressure approximately is 100+ age.

Diastolic pressure is the minimum pressure at the very end of ventricular diastole. It is the measure of constant stretch to which walls of the arteries are subjected. It is more important than systolic pressure because:

a. It is less fluctuating.
b. It is the constant load against which the heart has to work.
c. It is the pressure of peripheral resistance and depends mainly on the tone of the arteries.

Pulse pressure is the difference between the systolic and diastolic pressures. It is the rise in pressure caused by the ejection of blood into the aorta by ventricular contraction. It is a measure of stroke volume and compliance of arteries.

Mean arterial pressure is the average pressure present throughout the cardiac cycle. It is responsible for pushing the blood through the systemic circulatory system. It is equal to diastolic pressure + 1/3 pulse pressure.

Effect of Moderate Exercise on Blood Pressure

During exercise, there is a moderate increase in systolic blood pressure. This is due to an increase in cardiac output caused by an increased heart rate and myocardial contractility (stroke volume increases) due to increased sympathetic activity, and increased venous return. The increase in blood pressure is not proportionate to the increase in cardiac output because there is a reduction in total peripheral resistance. The effects of vasoconstriction in active regions is overcome by vasodilatation in active muscles. Hence the diastolic pressure at the pre-exercise level is slightly reduced. Pulse pressure is increased.

Result

Parameter	*At rest*	*After mild exercise*	*After moderate exercise*	*After severe exercise*
Systolic BP				
Diastolic BP				
Pulse pressure				
Mean arterial pressure				

QUESTIONS

1. Define (a) systolic blood pressure, (b) diastolic blood pressure, (c) pulse pressure, (d) mean arterial pressure.
2. Mention the different methods of determining blood pressure?

Student's Notes

3. What are the physiological factors affecting blood pressure?
4. What is the value of normal blood pressure? Give its acceptable range.
5. Comment on the mean values you obtained from your group.
   a. Is it within the normal range?
   b. Are there any members of your group who have abnormal values? Are there any attributable causes?
6. What are the possible sources of error in this experiment?
7. Why is the systolic pressure determined by the palpatory method lower than that determined by the auscultatory method?
8. Why is it important to first check the BP by the palpatory method always?
9. How are the sounds of Korotkoff produced?
10. What are the precautions to be taken while measuring blood pressure in:
    a. Children
    b. Obese individuals
11. Explain how the BP readings change in the following conditions. Explain the basis for these changes.
    a. When the arm is raised above the head
    b. If the cuff is applied to the thigh
12. While calculating the mean arterial pressure, what formula do we use and why?
13. Give 2 conditions when blood pressure is abnormally:
    a. Increased
    b. Decreased
14. Briefly describe 2 other methods of measuring blood pressure?
15. What is the physiological basis for postural hypotension?
16. What are the BP changes you observe during exercise in the subjects?
17. What are the changes in heart rate you observe after exercise? What is the physiological basis for these changes? How are they mediated?
18. Who first recorded the blood pressure?
19. Who invented the mercury manometer?
20. How is hypertension classified. What are their percentage.

BLOOD PRESSURE

Name: .... Age: ....

Sex: .... Occupation: ....

General Examination

Effect of Exercise on BP

Procedure	*Pulse (Rate per mm)*	*Systolic BP (mm Hg)*	*Diastolic BP (mm Hg)*	*Pulse pressure (mm Hg)*	*Mean arterial pressure DBP+ 1/3 PP (mm Hg)*
Before exercise					
After exercise					

Effect of Posture on BP

Procedure	*Pulse (Rate per mm)*	*Systolic BP (mm Hg)*	*Diastolic BP (mm Hg)*	*Pulse pressure (mm Hg)*	*Mean arterial pressure DBP+ 1/3 PP (mm Hg)*
Sitting					
Lying					
Standing					

Inference:

Student's Notes

Experiment 8: Electrocardiography

Aim

To record and analyze electrocardiogram (ECG) of a normal subject.

Requirements

Electrocardiograph, ECG leads (electrodes), ECG paper, straps and ECG jelly.

Description

Electrocardiograph

This is the equipment that can pick up, amplify and record from the body surface the electric potentials generated by the heart. Einthoven (1903) devised and used string galvanometer for this purpose. This instrument must be sensitive to potential changes of the order of microvolts and have a frequency response of 50–100 Hz. At present, transistors, amplifiers and cathode ray tubes are used for this purpose. Biopotentials are amplified to drive a galvanometer. Recording is obtained on a heat-sensitive paper using a hot stylus, an ink-writing pen or a photographic paper. Speed of the paper can be adjusted at 25 or 50 mm/sec. Using a polygraph or an oscilloscope; recording can be obtained at higher speeds. The sensitivity can be adjusted to 1 mV = 1 cm (or 2 cm or 0.5 cm).

Electrocardiogram

It is the graphic record of algebraic sum of action potentials developed during a cardiac cycle and recorded from the body surface: ECG paper has horizontal and vertical rulings at 1 mm distance. Every fifth line (5 mm) is thicker. At a paper speed of 25 mm/sec, 1 mm (vertical lines) = 40 msec. At a calibration of 1 cm = 1 mv, 1 mm (horizontal lines) = 0.1 mV.

ECG Leads

A lead or an electrode is a metal plate applied snugly over an appropriate body part. For better contact, saline or ECG jelly is applied after the skin surface is cleaned thoroughly. The leads are classified as following:

I. *Direct Leads*

Direct leads are applied directly to the heart during surgery or an experiment. An electrode can also be fixed on the tip of a catheter and introduce into the heart via a blood vessel. This is done for recording His bundle electrocardiogram (HBE).

II. *Indirect Leads*

1. *Esophageal leads:* Here, a miniature electrode is fixed on the tip of an esophageal catheter and positioned in esophagus so as to be close to cardiac chambers (e.g. posterior wall of right atrium). The lead is denoted by the letter E and a number indicates the distance of the electrode from the incisor teeth. For example, E20 indicates that the esophageal electrode is 20 cm from the incisor teeth.
2. *Bipolar limb leads:* These are leads I, II and III. Here, both the electrodes pick up the potentials from the body surface. The electrodes are attached to the right arm, left arm, and left foot as indicated in the Einthoven's triangle.
3. *Unipolar limb leads:* These are aVL, aVR and aVF. Here 'a' denotes augmented (i.e. aVR is 50% more amplitude than VR). 'V' denotes voltage and 'R', 'L' and 'F' indicatc that the exploring electrode on the right arm, left arm and left foot respectively. The another one electrode is connected to the right foot through a high resistance.

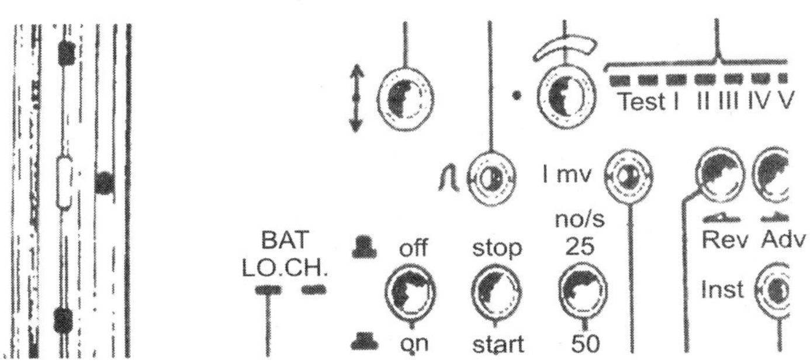

Fig. 8.1: Electrocardiograph

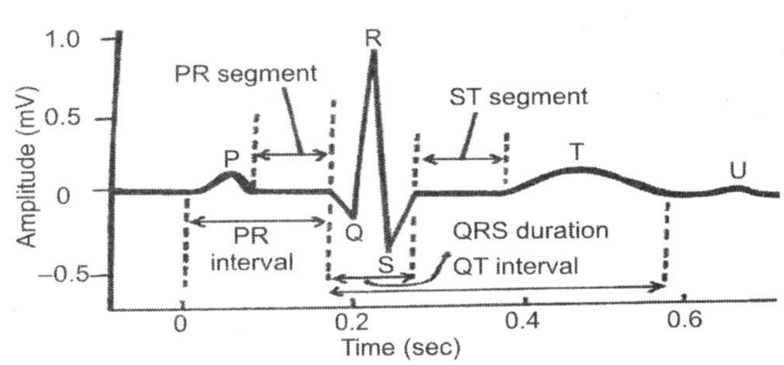

Fig. 8.2: Electrocardiogram

4. *Unipolar chest leads:* These are V1 to V6. Here, the passive or indifferent electrode is connected to Wilson terminal which is maintained at near zero potential and the exploring electrode is on the chest surface.
5. *Bipolar chest leads:* Here, one electrode is positioned on the chest wall as in V1 to V6 and the other electrode is on the right arm. Records obtained by bipolar chest leads are very similar to those obtained by unipolar chest leads. For routine electrocardiography, 12 leads (I, II, III, aVR, aVL, aVF and V1 to V6) are recorded and analyzed.

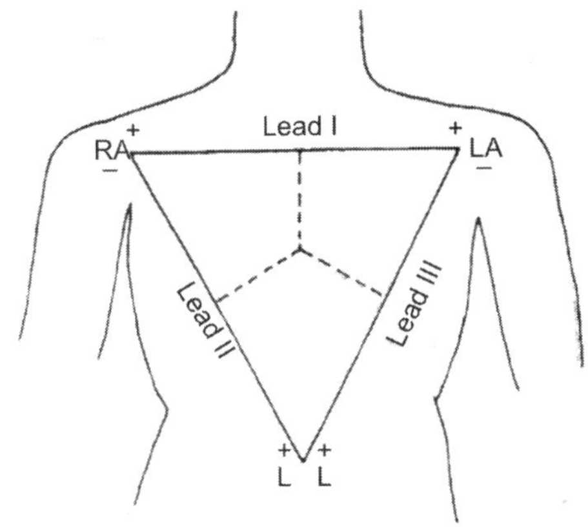

Fig. 8.3: Einthoven's triangle

Procedure

Before fixing the lead, clean the skin thoroughly and apply ECG jelly. The subject should lie down supine and completely relaxed to avoid muscle potentials. The right leg is earthed. Record in order of leads I, II, III, aVR, aVL, aVF and V1 to V6.

Calculation the heart rate (HR):

$$HR = \frac{60\ \text{seconds}}{\text{RR interval (in seconds)}}$$

At a paper speed of 25 mm/second,

$$HR = \frac{25 \times 60}{\text{RR interval in no. of small square on ECG paper}}$$

$$= \frac{1500}{\text{RR (mm)}}$$

$$= \frac{300}{\text{RR interval in no. of large squares on ECG paper}}$$

Calculation of Ventricular Vector (Mean Electrical Axis)

Calculate the net value of the QRS (R-S in mm) from leads I, II and III. Draw an equilateral triangle. From the midpoint of its each arm, mark in millimeters on the + and – sides. Draw vertical lines from the midpoints so that they meet at the midpoint of the triangle. Mark on each limb (lead) the net QRS values and draw vertical lines from these points. Let the lines meet at a point. Connect this point with the midpoint of the triangle. This gives the magnitude (depending on the length) and the direction (depending on the angle) of the net ventricular complex. Normal axis is about +600 (range: –30 to +110).

QUESTIONS

1. List the differences between action potential and ECG.
2. With the help of diagrams, show how various leads are connected for recording ECG.
3. Draw a normal lead II ECG and label it.
4. Measure and tabulate durations and amplitudes of various waves, intervals and segments from lead II of ECG.
5. Calculate QRS axis using Einthoven's triangle.
6. Name the physiological and pathological conditions that shift the ventricular axis to the left/right.
7. Calculate heart rate from the recorded ECG
8. Draw a diagram showing ECG, left ventricular pressure changes and heart sounds on the same time scale.
9. What is 'J' point?
10. What conditions cause ST elevation and ST depression?
11. What are the causes of tall T-waves and inverted T-waves?

Student's Notes

Experiment 9: Examination of Sensory System

Aim

To check the following sensations in the given subject:

1. Tactile sensibility—touch, localization, discrimination
2. Pain and temperature
3. Position and vibration sense
4. Stereognosis.

Procedure

The following tests are done with the subject's eyes closed.

Tactile Sensibility

This includes light touch, pressure, tactile localization and discrimination.

Light touch: Corresponding points of the different parts of the body on the two sides are touched with a wisp of cotton wool and the subject is asked to say whether he feels the sensation of touch.

Pressure touch is tested with the point of a finger or any blunt object.

Tactile localization: The subject is asked to localize the stimulus by indicating the exact position of the spot touched with eyes closed. Sensibility to touch may be altered in various ways.

1. If entirely abolished, it is called anaesthesia.
2. Partial loss is called hypoesthesia.
3. When touch produces painful irritating, tingling sensation it is referred to as hyperaesthesia.

Tactile discrimination: The two points of a compass are applied to the finger tips, arms and to the back of the subject. The minimum distance in millimetres at which the two points of the compass are felt separately is noted. There is a marked difference in the distances at which the two points of the compass are felt separately at the finger tip palmar surface of finger the forearm or middle of the back. Normally 2 mm of separation of the points can be recognized as two separate stimuli on the finger tips, 1 cm on the palmar surface and more in other area.

Pain

The sensation of superficial pain is examined by giving pricks with a steel pin to the different parts of the body. The subject is asked to describe the nature of sensation.

Deep pain is tested by pressing a muscle between thumb and index finger or the tendo-Achilles and the sensation felt is enquired about.

Absence of pain sensibility is termed as analgesia, partial loss is termed as hypoalgesia and an exaggerated sensibility is called as hyperalgesia.

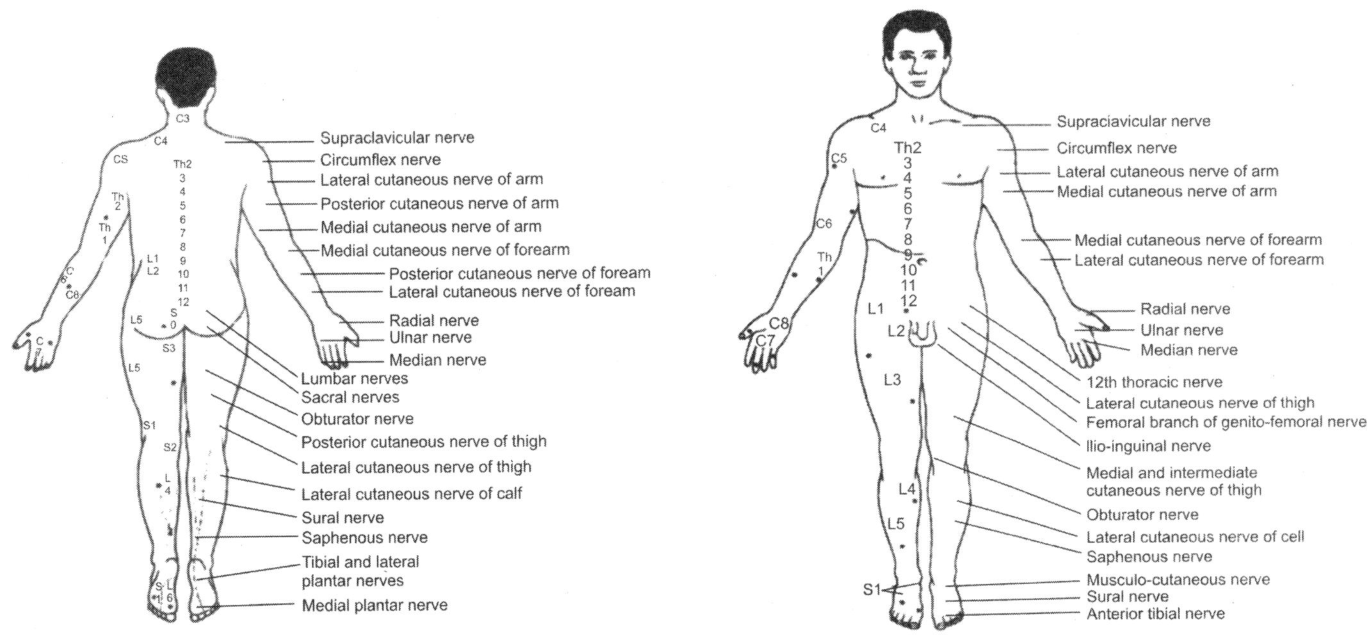

Fig. 9.1: Dermatomal patterns

Student's Notes

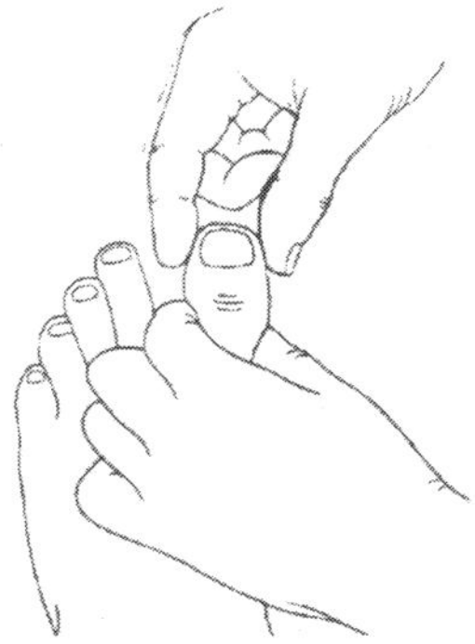

Fig. 9.2: Testing position sense

Temperature

In two test tubes, warm and cold water is taken. The test tubes are then applied to different parts of the body separately. The subject is asked to tell whether he feels warmth or cold. Test tube containing cold water is tested first may use ther moaestheriorneter.

Pour in cold water ⟷ Pour in cold water

Sense of Position and Passive Movement

With the eyes of the subject closed, one of his fingers flexed and extended passively. The subject is asked to say whether he felt any movement; if so, what movement it was. Involvement of 10° can be appreciated at all normal joints. In this way, different joints of the body are moved and the sense of passive movement are tested. The finger or a toe of the subject is moved up and down and is to be held there. The position of the part moved is enquired from the subject. Normally the subject would be able to appreciate the passive movements and the position of his limb. The subject may also be asked to imitate with the opposite limb or digit. The position of the limb is also tested.

Vibration

A vibrating tuning fork of 128 Hz is applied to the various bony prominences of the body and an enquiry is made regarding the sensation, felt by the subject. Normally, he would be able to feel the vibration. Usually, the tuning fork is placed on dorsum of great toe, lateral malleolus, dorsum of the finger and top of the acromion.

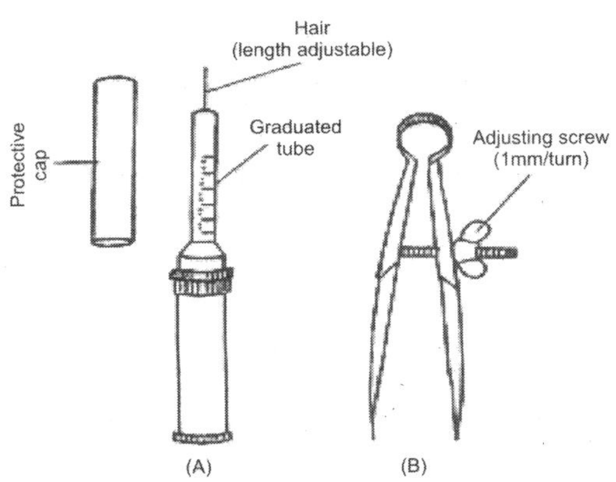

Fig. 9.3: An aesthesiometer (A) simple hair, (B) compass

Sterognosis

With the subject's eyes closed he is given some articles which are commonly used, e.g. coins, pens, etc. in his hand and he is asked to name them. Normally, he would be able to appreciate them with his eyes closed by their size, weight, shape, texture, temperature, etc. Loss of this power is known as astereognosis. The subject should use one hand only to feel the given object.

Abnormal Sensation

Paraesthesia is the various sensations experienced in the absence of any outward stimulus; there is a feeling of pins and needles, of numbness or insects crawling over the body.

Observation

Record your results in a tabular column.

QUESTIONS

1. What is epicritic and protopathic sensations?
2. What is proprioception? Name the receptors?
3. What is the receptor for pain, cold, hot, touch sensation?
4. What is pacinian corpuscles?
5. What is stereognosis?
6. Define analgesia, anaesthesia, hyperalgesia and hyperesthesia?
7. Name the tract carrying pain and touch sensation.
8. What is the Brodman's area number for primary sensory area and secondary sensory area?
9. What is tactile localization and discrimination?
10. Name the nucleus of the thalamus for conscious sensations.
11. Differentiate between fine and crude touch.
12. Can tuning fork with higher frequency (above 256 Hz)be used to test vibration sense?
13. Name few clinical conditions where vibration sense is lost.

Student's Notes

SENSORY SYSTEM

Name: .... Age: ....

Sex: .... Occupation: ....

General Examination

Higher function

Sensory System Examination

Prameters	*Upper limb* Right	*Upper limb* Left	*Lower limb* Right	*Lower limb* Left	*Others*
1. Touch					
Fine touch					
Crude touch					
Tactile localization					
Tactile discrimination (in mm)					
Palm					
Back					
Back					
Toes					
2. Pain					
Superficial					
Deep					
3. Temperature					
Cold					
4. Joint position sense					
Small joints					
Large joints					
5. Vibration sense					
6. Stereognosis					
7. Romberg's sign					

Inference:

Student's Notes

Experiment 10: Examination of Motor System

The motor system should be examined under the following aspects:

1. Bulk or nutrition of the muscles.
2. Tone of the muscles.
3. Strength of the muscles.
4. Reflexes
5. Co-ordination of movements
6. Involuntary movements

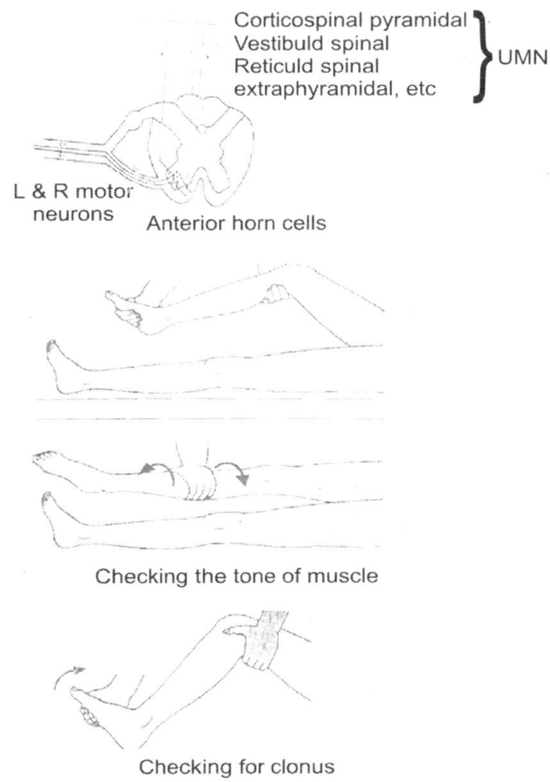

Fig. 10.1

Bulk of Muscles

Wasted and atrophic muscles are not only smaller but also softer and more flabbier than normal when they are contracted. Bulk of muscles is also assessed by measuring the circumference of the limbs with a tape at certain points with reference to definite bony landmarks and comparing on both sides.

The different muscles of the body are inspected and palpated and any wasting of musçles are to be noted. Similarly any contracture of the muscles are also to be observed. Muscle wasting and contracture are characteristic of poliomyelitis and muscular dystrophy.

Tone of the Muscles

Muscle tone is a state of tension or contraction found in healthy muscles. It is tested by passively moving the limbs at different joints and noting the resistance offered by the muscles during this process.

A. Hypertonia—increase in tone. It is of two types.
   1. Clasp knife I spastic rigidity—due to lesion in the corticospinal system:
   2. Cog-wheel/extrapyramidal rigidity—due to disease of the basal ganglia.

B. Hypotonia—decrease in tone, e.g. poliomyelitis.

Strength of the Muscles

Tested by asking the subject to carry out the action of muscle against resistance offered by examiner.

Testing Muscles of the Upper Limb

1. *Abductor pollicis brevis:* The subject is asked to abduct the thumb against resistance in a plane at right angle to palmar aspect of the index finger.
2. *Opponens pollicis:* The subject is asked to touch the tip of his little finger with the point of his thumb against resistance.
3. *First dorsal interosseous:* The subject is asked to abduct his index finger against resistance.
4. *Interosseus and lumbricals:* The subject is asked to flex the metacarpophalangeal joints and to extend the distal interphalangeal joints. The subject is also asked to abduct the finger. In ulnar nerve paralysis, "claw hand" deformity is produced. The first phalanges are over extended and the distal two are flexed. The fingers are slightly separated.
5. *Flexors of the fingers:* The subject is asked to squeeze the examiners index and middle finger.
6. *Flexors of the wrist:* The subject is asked to bring the tips of his fingers towards the front of the forearm.
7. *Extensor of the wrist:* The subject is asked to make a fist and the examiner tries to forcibly extend the wrist against the subjects effort to maintain this posture. Weakness or paralysis of extensor (wrist drop) occurs in radial nerve palsy.
8. *Brachioradialis:* The arm is placed midway between the prone and supine position and the subject is

Student's Notes

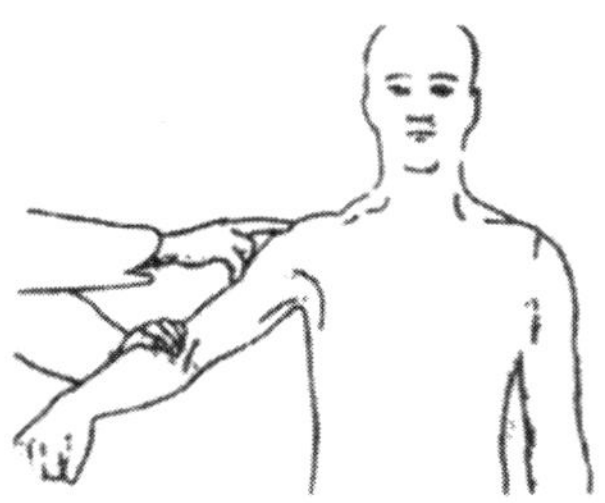

Testing the deltoid

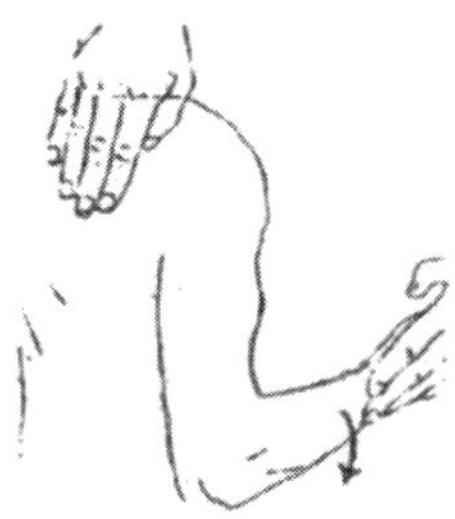

Testing the infraspinatus

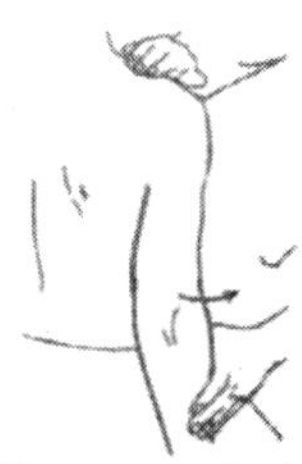

Testing the supraspinatus

Fig. 10.2

asked to bend the forearm against resistance. The muscle (if healthy) will stand out prominently at its upper part.

9. *Biceps:* The subject is asked to bend up the forearm against resistance with the forearm in full supination. The muscle will stand out clearly.
10. *Triceps:* The subject is asked to straighten out his flexed forearm against resistance.
11. *Supraspinatus:* The subject is asked to lift his arm straight at right angles to his side. The first 30° of this movement is carried out by the supraspinatus. The remaining 60° is by the deltoid.
12. *Deltoid:* The anterior and posterior fibers help to draw the abducted arm forwards and backwards respectively. The middle fibers abduct the shoulder.
13. *Infraspinatus:* The subject is asked to tuck his elbow into his side with the forearm flexed at right angle. He is then asked to rotate outwards against resistance. The elbow being held against the side throughout. The muscle can be seen and felt to contract.
14. *Pectorals:* The subject is asked to stretch his arms out in front of him and then clap his hands together while the examiner endeavors to hold them apart.
15. *Serratus anterior:* The subject is asked to push forward his hands against resistance such as wall. If there is paralysis of serratus anterior there would be 'winging' of the scapula.
16. *Latissimus dorsi:* The subject is asked to clasp his hands behind his back while the examiner standing behind the patient offer passive resistance to the down ward and backward movement.

Testing Muscles of the Trunk

Abdominal muscles: The subject lying in a spine position is asked to lift up his head from the pillow against resistance. In paralysis of the lower segment, the umbilicus moves upward, but when the upper segment is involved the umbilicus is pulled downwards. This is called as Beevors sign.

In weakness of the abdominal muscles, the patient would be unable to sit up in bed from the supine position without the aid of his arms. (Babinski's rising up sign.) Muscles of the back: The subject is asked to lie on his face and is asked to raise his head from the bed by extending the neck and back. The muscles of the back will standout prominently..

Trapezius: The patient is asked to shrug his shoulders against resistance.

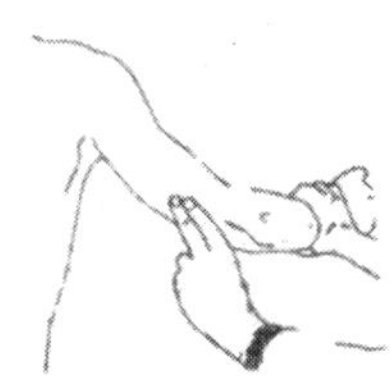

Testing the triceps

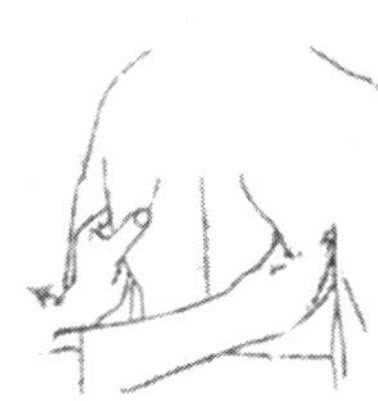

Testing the serratus anterior

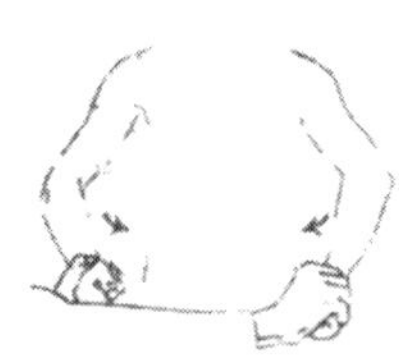

Testing the latissimus dorsi

Fig. 10.3

Student's Notes

Testing Muscles of the Lower Limb

Dorsi flexion and plantar flexion of the feet and toes are tested by asking the subject to elevate or depress the distal foot against resistance.

Extensors of the knee: The subject is asked to bend the knee. And then pressing the shin with the examiners hand the patient is asked to straighten it out again.

Flexors of the knee: The patient is asked to raise the leg up from the bed, the thigh being supported with the examiners left hand and the ankle with the right. The patient is then asked to bend his knee.

Extensors of the hip: With the knee being extended, the patient's foot is lifted off the bed. The subject is asked to push it down against resistance.

Flexors of the thigh: With the leg extended the patient is asked to raise his leg of the bed against resistance.

Abductors of thigh: The subject's legs are placed together. He is then asked to separate them against resistance.

Adductors of the thigh: Abduct the limbs and ask the subject to bring them back to midline against resistance.

Rotators of the thigh: With the lower limb extended on the bed, the patient is asked to roll it outwards or inwards against resistance.

Grading of Weakness

Grade 0—Complete paralysis
Grade 1—Flicker of contraction only

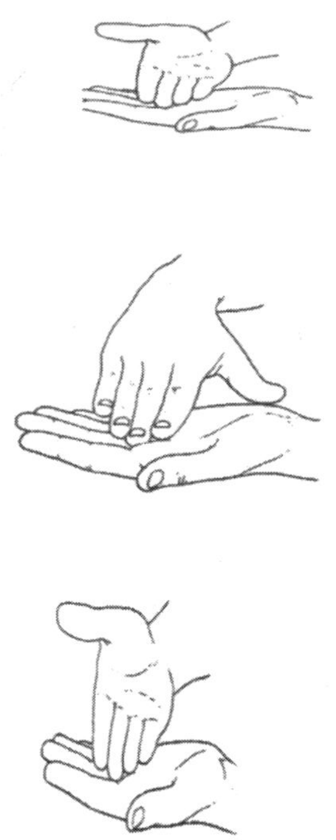

Fig. 10.4: Looking for dysdiabochokinesis

Grade 2—Power detectable only when gravity is excluded by appropriate adjustment.
Grade 3—The limb can be bent against the force of gravity, but not against the examiner's resistance.
Grade 4—There is some degree of weakness, usually described as poor, fair, or moderate strength.
Grade 5—Normal power.

Patterns of Weakness

Hemiplegia: Paralysis of one side of the body, especially of the arm and leg and usually of the jaw

Paraplegia: Paralysis of both legs.

Quadriplegia: All four limbs are paralysed

Reflexes

1. Superficial reflexes
2. Deep reflexes.
3. Visceral reflexes.

Grading of Deep Reflexes

0. Absent,
1. Present (as a normal ankle jerk)
2. Brisk (as a normal knee jerk)
3. Very brisk
4. Clonus.

Coordination of Movement

By coordination, it is meant the smooth recruitment, interaction and cooperation of separate muscles or groups of muscles in order to accomplish a definite motor act.

If coordination is imperfect, ataxia is said to be present.

The coordination of groups of muscle is a function of various factors, among which are different impulses coming from the muscle spindles and joint receptors, cerebellar function and the state of tone of the muscles.

Test for Coordination

In the upper limbs:

1. The subject is asked to touch his nose first with open eyes and then with the closed eyes repeatedly (finger-nose test).
2. The subject is asked to touch his nose first and then the examiner's forefinger with his index finger. The same tests are done with the eyes closed (finger-finger-nose test).
3. The subject is asked to flex his elbows to a right angle and then alternately supinate and pronate his forearms as rapidly as possible. In dysdiadokinesia (a sign of cerebellar ataxia), the movements are slow,

Student's Notes

awkward and incomplete and often impossible after a few attempts. In addition, the rhythm of the movement in characteristically irregular.

4. Coordination can also be assessed by everyday movements like dressing or undressing, handling a book or picking up pins or threading a needle.

In the lower limbs:

1. The subject is asked to walk along a straight line. If incoordination is present, he will soon deviate to one side or the other.
2. *Knee-heel test:* The subject is asked to lie in bed and to lift one leg high in the air and to place the heel of his leg on the opposite knee and then to slide the heel down his shin towards the ankle. The test should be performed with the eyes open. In cerebellar ataxia, a characteristic, irregular side to side series of error in the speed and direction of' movement occurs. Heel knee test. Also called heel-shin-ankle test.
3. The subject is asked to draw a large circle in the air with his great toe. The circles should be drawn smoothly and accurately and the subject is asked to put a dot in the centre.
4. *Rhomberg's sign:* This test is for loss of position sense. It is not a test of cerebellar function. The subject is asked to stand with his feet close together and if he can do this, he is then asked to close his eyes. If Rhomberg's sign is present, as soon as his eyes are closed he begins to sway about or may even fall to the same side.

With defective position sense in the legs, as in tabes dorsalis (where posterior column is affected) or sensory neuropathy, the patient is unable to maintain his posture without the aid of vision. Patient with labyrinthine or cerebellar lesions do not show instability in this test.

Gait

To observe gait, the legs are adequately exposed and freed of constricting clothing and the feet bare. The subject is asked to walk away from the observer, to turn round at a given point and then to come towards him again. Certain points are to be noted.

1. Whether the subject could walk at all? If he could.
2. Whether he could walk in a straight line or deviated to one side or the other.
3. If the subject deviates to one side, the side of deviation is noted.

During examination of the gait, care is taken to see that the abnormal gait is not due to some surgical cause or to any local disease of the joint, e.g. osteoarthritis of the hip.

Well-recognized abnormal types of gait are:

1. Spastic gait or the hemiplegic gait. This type of gait is seen in hemiplegic patient.
2. Stamping' gait occurs during sensory ataxia. This gait is seen in tabes dorsalis.
3. 'Reeling, or 'drunken mans' gait occurs in cerebellar ataxia.
4. Festinant gait is seen in Parkinson's disease.
5. Waddling gait is seen in muscular dystrophy and myopathies.
6. High stepping gait is seen in weakness' of extensor muscles of the feet, e.g. in common peroneal nerve palsy.

Involuntary Movements

The involuntary movements occur either at rest or during voluntary movement.

Most are due to diseases of the basal ganglia and extrapyramidal system. The different involuntary movements are:

1. Epilepsy
2. Myoclonus
3. Tremors
   a. Fine tremors: Seen in anxiety, hyperthyroidism
   b. Coarse tremors
      i. Intentional tremor seen in cerebellar diseases.
      ii. Un intentional tremor seen in Parkinsonism.
   c. Hysterical—intentional
4. Athetosis
5. Chorea
6. Hemiballisimus
7. Tics.

Speech

Speech is higher function. The subject is asked to repeat a sentence put forth by the examiner and the pattern of speech is observed. Certain common disorders of speech are:

- Aphasia—absence of speech.
- Dysphasia—disturbance of speech.
- Aphasia and dysphasia are usually associated with higher centre lesion.
- Dysarthria—difficulty in articulation of speech.
- Dysarthria is usually associated with lesion in the phonation apparatus.

QUESTIONS

1. Define muscle tone in physiological terms.
2. Distinguish between spasticity and rigidity (types of hypertonia). Mention in which condition each occurs.

Student's Notes

3. Define: Hemiparesis, hemiplegia, paraplegia, quadriplegia.
4. Describe 2 tests of co-ordination (other than those mentioned in your record)
5. What is Hypertrophy, hyperplasia and atrophy of muscles?
6. What is rigidity? Give example.
7. How do you grade the power of muscles?
8. What is the normal grade?
9. Which is the major descending motor tract?
10. Name some extrapyramidal tracts.
11. Which is the primary motor area of the cortex?
12. What is paralysis and paresis?
13. When does winging of scapula occurs?
14. What is saturday night paralysis?
15. What is chorea? Give examples.
16. What is athetosis? Give examples.
17. What is hemiballismus? Give examples.
18. What is parkinsonism?
19. What is tremor? Classify with examples.
20. What happens when radial and ulnar nerves are paralysed?
21. Name some abnormal gaits and mention the conditions where it occurs.
22. What is a stretch reflex?
23. What is Jendrassik's manoeuvre?
24. What are the different aspects of motor functions that are assessed while examining the motor system.
25. How do you measure the bulk of the muscles in the upper and lower limbs. Name four bony landmarks.
26. How do you estimate the strength of the intrinsic muscles of hand.
27. How do you assess the strength of the trunk muscles.
28. How do you assess the strength of extensors and flexors of the knee and thigh?

Student's Notes

MOTOR SYSTEM

Name: .... Sex: ....

Age: .... Occupation: ....

General Examination

Higher Function

Bulk of muscles (in cm)	*Right*	*Left*
Upper limb 1. Upper arm 2. Forearm		
Lower limb 1. Thigh 2. Leg		

Tone of the muscle	*Right*	*Left*
Upper limb At small joints At large joints		
Lower limb At small joints At large joints		

Strength power of the muscle	*Grade*	
	Right	*Left*
1. Abductor pollicis brevis 2. Opponens pollicis 3. First dorsal interossei 4. Interrossei and lumbricals 5. Flexors of the fingers 6. Flexors of the wrist 7. Extensors of wrist 8. Brachioradialis 9. Biceps 10. Triceps		

IV. Reflexes

V. Coordination of muscles

VI. Involuntary movements

VII. Gait

Inference:

Student's Notes

Experiment 11: Reflexes

Aim

To elicit the superficial, deep and visceral reflexes on the subject.

Requisites

1. Knee hammer
2. Torch light
3. Cotton swab

The various reflexes are elicited under the following headings.

SUPERFICIAL REFLEXES

On stimulation of a particular part of skin or mucous membrane, contraction of certain muscles results. A lesion at any part of the reflex path causes the reflexes to disappear, e.g. anaesthesia of skin, disease of sensory fibers or posterior nerve root, changes in grey matter of the cord, lesions of motor fibers or muscles. In UMN lesion, the reflexes are affected on the paralysed side.

1. Conjunctival Reflex: (Aff- V, Eff- VII Cranial)

The conjunctiva of the eye is touched with a wisp of cotton. *Observation:* Closure of eyelids.

2. Corneal Reflex: (Aff- V, Eff- VII Cranial)

The sclerocorneal junction is touched with a wisp of cotton. *Observation:* Closure of eyelids.

3. Pupillary Reflexes: (Aff- H, Eff- III Cranial)

a. ***Light reflex:***
   i. *Direct light reflex:* The subject is asked to sit in a dimly lit room. A beam of bright light using a torch is thrown on one eye. *Observation:* Constriction of the pupil on the illuminated eye. Similarly the other eye is tested.
   ii. *Indirect light reflex (consensual light reflex):* A beam of light is thrown on one eye the other eye is observed. *Observation:* Constriction of the pupil on the opposite side.

b. ***Accommodation reflex:***
   The subject is asked to look at a distant object. The size of the pupil is noted. Immediately the subject is asked to look at the finger placed in front of his eyes. Pupillary constriction is observed.

4. Cub Spinal Reflex: (Cervical Symp)

The skin on the side of the neck is stroked or pinched. *Observation:* Dilatation of the pupil.

5. Abdominal Reflex: (T6 –T12)

The skin of the anterior abdominal wall is gently stroked on the four quadrants with the sharp end of the knee hammer obliquely. *Observation:* Contraction of the muscles on the side stroked.

6. Cremastric Reflex: (L1, L2)

The medial side of the thigh is stroked in the male subject. *Observation:* Elevation of the testicle or the scrotal sac of the same side.

7. Anal Reflex: (S3, S4)

The skin around the anus is stroked.
Observation: Contraction of the anal sphincter

8. Plantar Reflex: (L5, S1)

The outer edge of the sole of the foot is stroked gently from the heel towards the ball of the little toe and

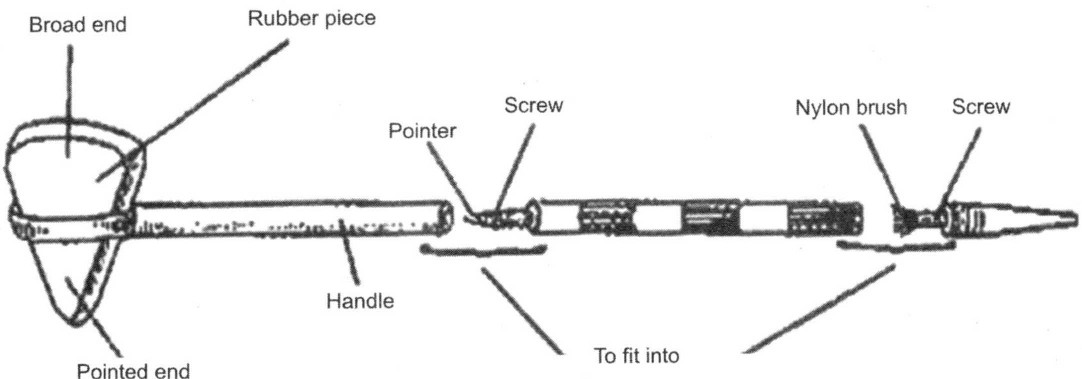

Fig. 11.1: Knee hammer

Student's Notes

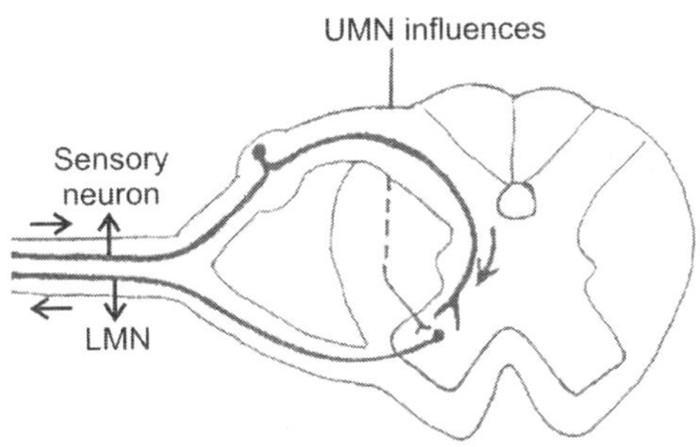

Fig. 11.2: Reflex arc

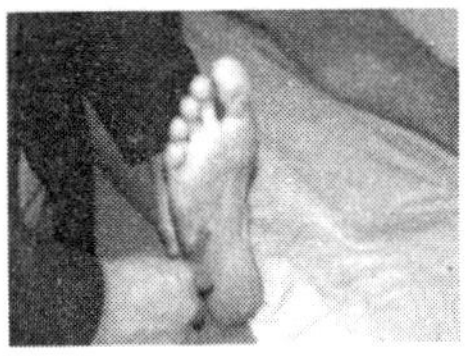

Plantar reflex

continued medially up to the ball of the great toe in one stroke with the blunt end of a knee hammer.

Observation: Plantar flexion of the great toe and the other four toes. flexed and draw together.

Babinski's sign: Seen in upper motor neuron lesion. In this condition, there is dorsiflexion of the great toe and fanning of other toes. It is also seen in infants below one year.

DEEP REFLEXES

When the tendon of a lightly stretched muscle is struck, a single sharp blow with soft rubber hammer, the muscle contracts briefly, this is tendon or stretch reflex.

1. Jaw Jerk: (Cranial V)

The subject is asked to keep his mouth half opened. A finger is placed on chin of the subject and the finger struck with a knee hammer.

Observation: Closure of the mouth.

2. Biceps Jerk: (C5, C6)

The elbow of the subject is slightly flexed. The examiner's thumb is placed over the biceps tendon and the thumb struck with a knee hammer.

Observation: Contraction of the biceps.

3. Triceps Jerk: (C6, C7)

The elbow of the subject is flexed and the forearm is allowed to rest across the subject's chest. The triceps tendon just above the olecranon is tapped gently with a knee hammer.

Observation: Contraction of triceps.

4. Supinator Jerk: (Brachioradialis jerk) (C5, C6)

The elbow of the subject is gently flexed and the forearm half pronated. The tendon overlying the radial styloid process is gently tapped with a knee hammer.

Observation: Contraction of the brachioradialis muscle.

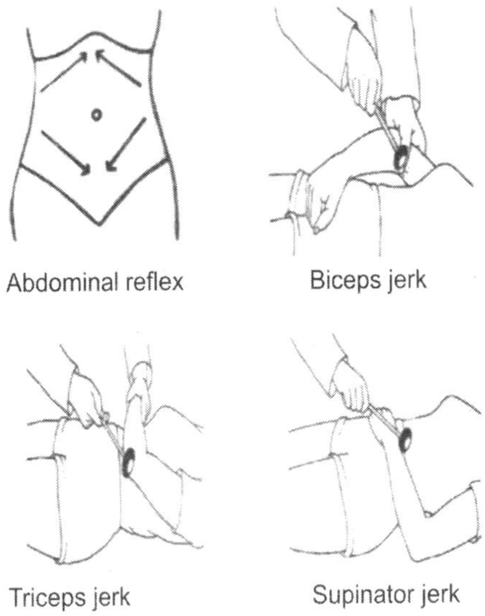

Fig. 11.3

5. Knee Jerk: (L2, L3)

The subject is allowed to be seated on a stool with one leg crossed over the other and hanging loosely. Examiner's hand is placed over the quadriceps muscle and the patellar tendon is gently tapped with a knee hammer. Observation: A forward kick of the leg would be observed due to contractions of the quadriceps muscle.

When the subject is lying supine the knee in supported, with the left hand and the patellar tendon is tapped.

Patellar clonus: With the leg fully extended at the knee joint, the patella is ripped between the thumb and the other fingers and pushed upwards. Observation: In a normal person, there may be a few contractions which immediately relaxes. In upper motor neuron lesion, sustained contractions may be seen.

6. Ankle Jerk: (SI, S2)

The subject is asked to sit on a stool with the leg crossed and with the foot slightly doriflexed by the examiner so as to apply slight tension on tendo-Achilles. The tendo-Achilles is tapped with a knee hammer. Observation: Contraction of calf muscles with plantar flexion.

Ankle clonus: The subject's knee is bent slightly and supported with left hand. The forefoot is grasped with the hand and suddenly dorsiflexed.

Student's Notes

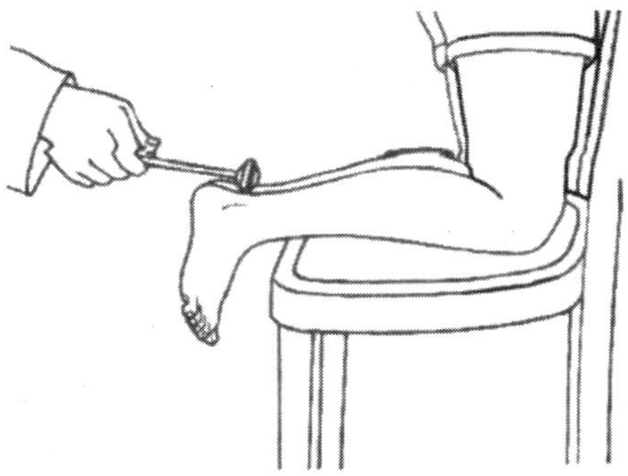

Ankle jerk–kneeling posture

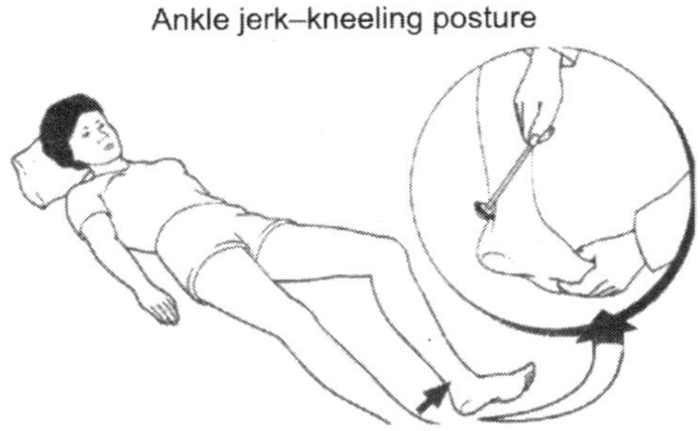

Ankle jerk–supine posture

Fig. 11.4

Observation: Interrmittent jerking movement can be observed which would be persistent in upper motor neuron lesion.

Grading of Reflexes

0—Absent
1—Present (as a normal ankle jerk)
2—Present (as a normal knee jerk) (Brisk)
3—Very brisk
4—Clonus.

VISCERAL REFLEXES

1. Defaecation Reflex

The subject was questioned about his bowel habits to rule out incontinence.

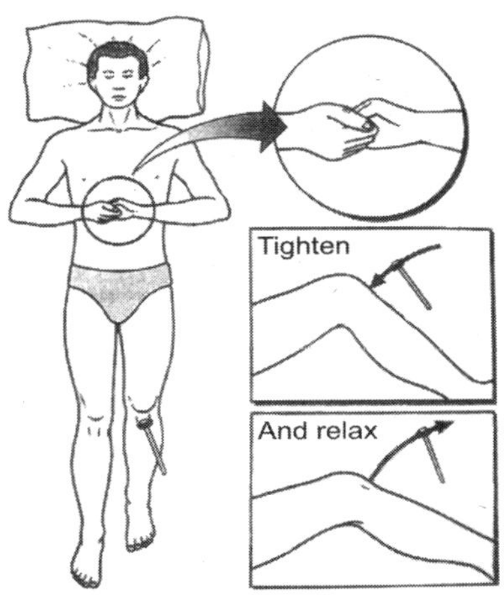

Fig. 11.5

2. Micturition Reflex

The subjects is questioned about his micturition habits to rule our bladder incontinence.

3. Swallowing Reflex (Deglutition Reflex)

The subject is questioned about.
i. Any difficulty in swallowing
ii. Nasal regurgitation of food during swallowing.

Reinforcement Technique (Jendrassik's Maneuver)

In healthy, the knee jerk is hardly seen or entirely absent. But in case of other tendon reflexes, sometimes it may be necessary to apply reinforcement—Jendrassik's manoeuvre. It is done by asking the subject to make a strong voluntary muscular effort such as hooking the fingers of the two hands together and pulling them apart. Reinforcement acts by increasing the excitability of anterior horn cells and by increasing the sensibility of the muscle spindle to stretch.

Abnormal Tendon Reflex

Hyporeflexia—diminished or absent tendon reflexes. Seen in lower motor tendon lesion, e.g. tabes dorsalis, poliomyelitis. Hyper-reflexia—exaggerated tendon reflexes.

Occurs in upper motor neuron lesion, anxious individuals, thyrotoxicosis, tetanus.

In cerebellar disease, the reflexes have a pendular quality.

Result:

QUESTIONS

1. Define a reflex?
2. Draw and label a reflex arc?
3. How will you grade a reflex?
4. List the differences between the upper motor neuron lesions and lower motor neuron lesions?
5. What is clonus?
6. What is Babinski's sign?
7. Give the different classification of reflexes?
8. What is Jendrassik's maneuver? Give its importance?
9. What is the root value of knee jerk, biceps jerk and ankle jerk?
10. What is crossed extensor reflex?
11. What is the root value of abdominal and plantar reflex?
12. How is the reflexes examination going to be useful to the physician?

Student's Notes

REFLEXES

Name: ....
Age: ....
Sex: ....
Occupation: ....

General Examination
Higher Functions

Superficial reflex	*Right*	*Left*	*Root value*
1. Conjunctival reflex			
2. Corneal reflex			
3. Pupillary reflex			
(i) Direct light reflex			
(ii) Indirect light reflex			
4. Accommodation reflex			
5.Upper abdominal reflex			
6. Lower abdominal reflex			
7. Plantar reflex			

Deep Reflex	*Right*	*Left*	*Root value*
1. Jaw jerk			
2. Biceps jerk			
3. Triceps jerk			
4. Brachioradialis/supinator jerk			
5. Knee jerk			
6. Ankle jerk			

Visceral Reflexes

1. Defaecation reflex
2. Micturition reflex
3. Swallowing reflex

Inference:

Student's Notes

Experiment 12: Examination of Cranial Nerves I to VI

Aim

To examine the cranial nerves I, II, III, IV, V and VI.

I. OLFACTORY NERVE

Anatomy

Serves the sense of smell, receptors are found in the mucous membrane of the roof of the nasal cavity. From here the fibres pass via the cribriform plate of the ethmoid bone to the glomeruli of the olfactory bulb and later it reaches the cerebral cortex to end in the uncus of the parahippocampal gyrus.

Tests for Smell

The sense of smell is tested in each nostril separately with eyes closed. Substances like oil of peppermint, oil of clove, tincture of asafoetida are used. Irritating substances like ammonia are avoided since it would partially stimulate the trigeminal nerve.

Abnormalities

- Anosmia—loss of sensation of smell as seen in cases of meningitis, fracture of anterior cranial fossa, etc.
- Parosmia—perverted smell as seen in head injuries.
- Hyposmia—decrease in a perception of smell.

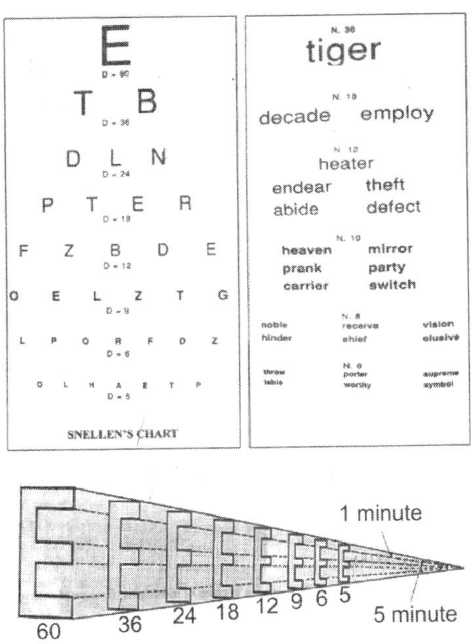

Fig. 12.1: Principle behind Snellen's chart test

II. OPTIC NERVE

Anatomy

The receptors for visions are the rods and cones of retina. From here, the fibres pass backward as the optic nerve. The two optic nerve then forms the optic chiasma. Fibres of the optic nerve continue as optic radiations and end in the striate area of the occipital cortex.

Tests

1. Acuity of vision
2. Field of vision
3. Colour vision
4. Pupillary response.

Acuity of Vision

1. *Test for distant vision:* Using Snellen's test types, each eye is tested separately. A chart containing letters of different sizes is kept at a distance of 6 meters from the subject. Under each line on the chart is a number which indicates the distances at which the line should be read. Visual acuity is determined by the formula V=d/D where 'd' is the distance at which the letters are read and 'D' is the distance at which they should be read.
   When 'V' is less than 1/60, other tests are done like
   i. Finger counting test
   ii. Hand movement test
   iii. Perception or no perception of light.
2. *Test for near vision:* This is assessed by using Jaeger's chart which has letters of different sizes. The smallest print is 0.5 mm. The near vision is recorded as the smallest type which the subject can read comfortably.

Field of Vision

This represents that portion of space in which other objects are visible while fixing the gaze on a particular object.

1. *Confrontation method:* The test is done first for each eye individually. The subject and the examiner is seated at an arm's distance. (If the subject's left eye is to be tested, the subject should close his right eye and the examiner his left eye, so that the subject's left eye and the examiner's right eye confront each other). The examiner holds the'index finger of his outstretched left hand to a plane midway between him and the

Student's Notes

patient. The finger is brought nearer to the midline until the examiner first perceives the moving finger. The subject is asked if he is also able to be see finger. If he fails to do so, the finger is brought nearer until he sees them. The field is tested in each eye separately in every direction—upwards, downwards, to right and to left—using the extent of the examiner's own field for comparison.

2. *Instrumental method:* Using perimeter. Abnormalities in the field of vision:
   1. Central scotoma—loss of vision confined to the centre of the field.
   2. Hemianopia—loss of vision in one-half of visual field.
      a. Heteronymous—same half of the both fields are affected.
         i. Binasal hemianopia—loss of vision in the nasal field in both eyes.
         ii. Bitemporal hemianopia—loss of vision in the temporal field in both eyes.
      b. Homonymous hemianopia
         i. Right homonymous hemianopia—right half of field of each eye is affected.
         ii. Left homonymous hemianopia—left half of each eye is affected.
   3. Quadrantanopia—loss of vision in a quadrant of the visual field.

Colour Vision

a. Holmgren's wool test
b. Ishihara's pseudoisochromatic charts. (*see* color plate)

Pupillary Response

It is dealt with under next section.

III, IV AND VI, OCULOMOTOR, TROCHLEAR AND ABDUCENT NERVES

Oculomotor Nerve Supplies

i. Extraocular muscles other than supplied by IV and VI cranial nerves.
ii. Sphincter pupillae
iii. Muscles of accommodation
iv. Levator palpabrae superioris

Edinger-Westphal nucleus supplies parasympathetic fibre to ciliary muscles and iris.

Trochlear nerve supplies superior oblique (SO_4)
Abducent nerve supplies lateral rectus. (LR_6)

Examination of the Extra-ocular-Muscles Movement

The superior and inferior recti act as elevators and depressors alone when the eye is in abduction. The obliques act similarly when the eye is in adduction. (Superior oblique act as depressors of the eye and inferior oblique act as elevators).

Supranuclear Lesion

1. Loss of conjugate movements of eyes
2. Skew deviation of eyes
3. Nystagmus

Infranuclear lesion: There is paralysis of individual muscles.

Paralysis of III N: There is ptosis or drooping of eyelid. The eyeball is displaced downward and outward. The pupil is dilated and there is loss of accommodation.

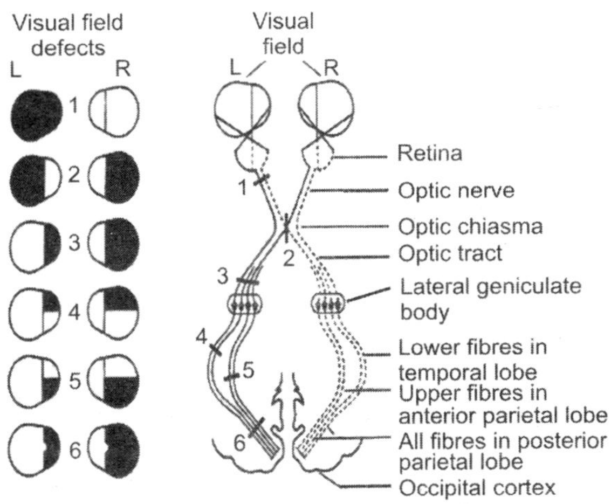

Fig. 12.3: Visual pathway and defects

Paralysis of IV N: Impaired downward movement. Eyeball rotated outwards due to unopposed action of inferior rectus when attempting to look downwards and diplopia below the horizontal plane.

Paralysis of VI N: Inability to move the eye outwards and diplopia on looking in that direction. Some times convergent squint due to unopposed action of medial rectus.

Examination of the Pupil

1. Size—compare both sides.
2. Shape—may be irregular due to adhesion of iris to lens following iritis.
3. Mobility.
   a. *Reaction to light:*
      i. Direct light reflex. There would be constriction of the pupil when a bright light is shown in that eye.

Student's Notes

ii. Indirect or consensual light reflex. When light is shown in one eye there will be constriction of the pupil of the opposite eye even when a hand or a book is placed between the eyes. This is due to crossing of fibres in the optic chiasma.

b. *Accommodation reflex:* When a person seeing a distant object is asked to focus on a near object, accommodation occurs. Together with accommodation there is miosis and convergence of the eyes.

Argyll Robertson pupil: Seen in neurosyphilis. In this condition, the lesion is in the pretectal region of mesencephalon. Accommodation reflex is present whereas the light reflex is absent.

V. TRIGEMINAL NERVE

Sensory pathway: From trigeminal (Gasserian) ganglion, the fibres enter the lateral surface of pons about its middle. Fibres for touch and postural sensibility terminate in large nucleus on pons (lateral to motor nucleus).

Fibres for pain and thermal sensation enter the descending or bulbospinal tract which extends up to C2 level and ascends in medial lemniscus.

The fibres arise from 3 divisions:

1. Ophthalmic
2. Maxillary
3. Mandibular

The mandibular division supplies parasympathetic fibres to the salivary glands.

Motor Pathway

Originates from the small nucleus medial to sensory nucleus. It emerges from the side of pons and passes inferior to trigeminal ganglion and joins the mandibular division to supply muscles of mastication namely masseter and temporalis.

Tests for Sensation

1. To test for cutaneous sensation.
2. To test for corneal reflex and conjunctival reflex.
3. To test for palatal reflex.

Tests for Motor Functions

1. The subject is asked to clench the teeth. The prominence of the masseter and temporalis is to be felt.

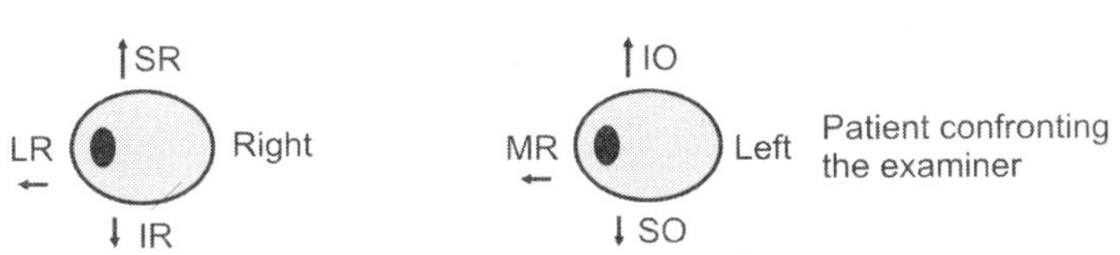

Fig. 12.4: Examination of the extraocular muscles movement

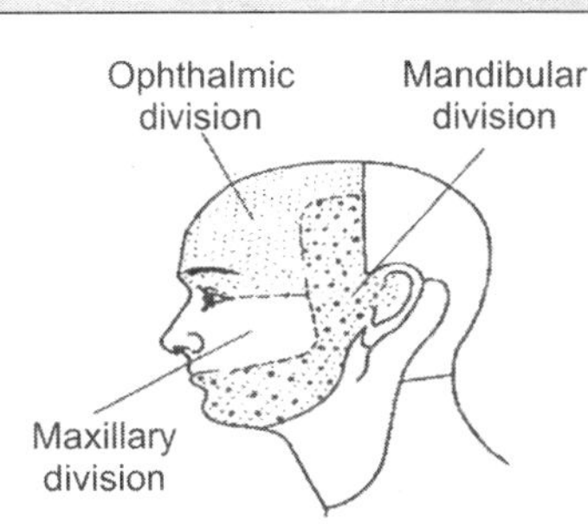

Fig. 12.5: Trigeminal nerve—sensory distribution

2. The subject is asked to open the mouth—In paralysis of the motor division of trigeminal nerve, the jaw is deviated to the paralysed side due to action of pterygoid muscle.

Lesion of Trigminal Nerve

1. Loss of sensation of skin and mucous membrane of jaw and nasopharynx.
2. Salivary, buccal and lacrimal secretion decreases.
3. Trophic ulcers in mouth, nose and cornea.
4. Weakness of muscles of mastication.

Observation: (write down you observations as directed in the class)

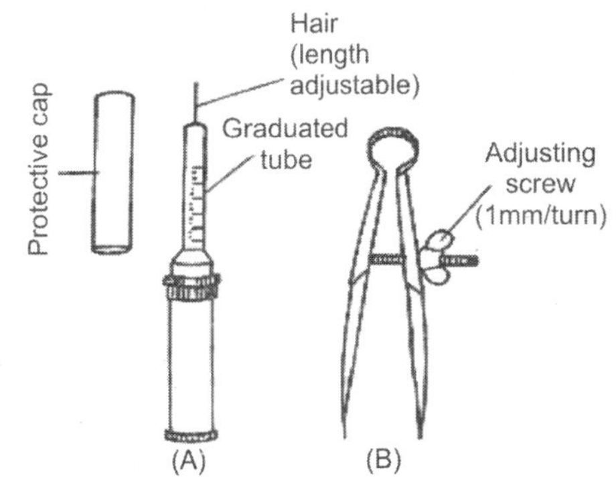

Fig. 12.6: An aesthesiometer (A) simple hair, (B) compass

QUESTIONS

1. Define anosmia, hyperosmia and parosmia. Mention the conditions in which these occur.
2. List the effects of various lesions in the visual pathway.
3. What is colour blindness? What are the types of the colour blindness? How is it transmitted in man?
4. How are supranuclear (UMN) and infranuclear (LMN) lesions of 3rd, 4th and 6th nerves differentiated?
5. What are the effects of lesions of the 5th nerve?
6. Describe Argyll Robertson pupil.
7. What is Horner's syndrome?
8. What are the receptors involved in colour vision?

Student's Notes

9. Why NH_3 is not used for smell test?
10. What is the instrument used for smell test? Olfactometer, Zwardimeter?
11. Define visual acquity and visual field. How is it tested?
12. What are the tests for colour vision?
13. What is blind spot?
14. What is the cause for indirect light reflex?
15. What is squint/strabismus?
16. What is cataract?
17. What are the manifestation of vitamin 'A' deficiency? Xerosis, Bitot's spots, nyctalopia keratomalacia.
18. What are muscles of mastication?
19. Which cranial nerve is commonly affected by increase in intracranial pressure?
20. What is glaucoma? Types and how is it tested?
21. What is the afferent nerve and efferent nerve for corneal reflex?
22. What are the divisions of 5th cranial nerve?
23. How will you test the motor function of the 5th nerve?

Student's Notes

CRANIAL NERVES I TO VI

Name: .... Age: ....
Sex: .... Occupation: ....

General Examination

Build and nutrition ....
Pallor ....
Lymphadenopathy ....
Pedal edema ....
Arterial pulse ....
BP ....
Temp ....
Higher functions
- Handedness
- Intelligence
- Consciousness
- Orientation
- Memory
- Emotion
- Behaviour
- Speech

Clubbing ....
Icterus ....
Cyanosis ....

Cranial Nerve I

No history of cold or nasal block

	Right nostril	*Left nostril*
Nicotine in solution		
Peppermint oil		
Clove oil		
Tincture of asafoetida		

Cranial Nerve II

	Distant vision (Snellen's)	*Near vision (Jaeger's)*
Visual acquity		
Right eye		
Left eye		

Field of Vision

	Superior	*Inferior*	*Medial*	*Lateral*
Right eye				
Left eye				

Colour Vision

Right eye:
Left eye:

Student's Notes

Pupillary Response (See Below)
Cranial Nerve III, IV, Vl
Pupils:

	Right eye	*Left eye*
Size		
Shape		
Direct light reflex		
Indirect light reflex		
Accommodation reflex		

Ocular movements:

	Right eye	*Left eye*
Action		
Adduction		
Abduction		
Elevation while adducted		
Depression while adducted		
Elevation while abducted		
Depression while abducted		

Cranial Nerve V
No history of loss of sensation in mouth or ulcers in mouth, nose and cornea

General sensations	*Ophthalmic division*		*Maxillary division*		*Mandibular division*	
	Right	*Left*	*Right*	*Left*	*Right*	*Left*
Touch						
Pain						
Vibration						
Temperature						
Tactile localization						
Tactile discrimination						

Reflexes:

	Right eye	*Left eye*
Corneal reflex		
Conjunctival reflex		

Sneeze reflex:
Motor function
Closure of the mouth:
Open the mouth:
Clench the teeth:
Jaw jerk:

Report:
Cranial nerves I to VI of the given subject were examined and found to be normal.

Student's Notes

Experiment 13: Examination of Cranial Nerves VII to XII

Aim

To examine the cranial nerves VII, VIII, IX, X, Xl and XII.

VII. FACIAL NERVE

Anatomy

From facial nucleus (situated lateral to abducent) fibers wind round the abducent nucleus and emerge medial to vestibulocochlear nerve. In close contact with the VIII nerve, it enters the auditory meatus. During its course in the temporal bone, it gives off a branch to stapedius muscle. It is joined by chorda tympani which contains taste fibres of the anterior two-thirds of tongue at the geniculate ganglion. It emerges at a point opposite the junction of the anterior border of the mastoid process and spreads to supply the facial muscles. Facial nerve is a motor nerve. It supplies all the muscles of the face and scalp except levator palpebrae superioris. It also supplies platysma.

Pathway for taste: From anterior two-thirds of the tongue, the fibres pass from lingual nerve to chorda tympani and through the geniculate ganglion of the facial nerve into medulla oblongata (sometimes passes in maxillary division of V nerve).

From the nucleus of tractus solitarius, the fibres pass to the thalamus and then to the temporal part of post-central gyrus and to amygdala.

Tests for Taste

1. The subject is asked to protrude his tongue. The test substance used are sugar and salt.

The substance is placed on the tongue and the subject is asked to indicate the perception of the taste without withdrawing the tongue. After each test, the mouth must be rinsed. Quinine and citric acid are used to test bitter and sour tastes. Quinine test must be applied last.

1. The subject is asked for abnormal tastes or hallucinations of taste.

   Abnormalities: Ageusia—loss of taste sensation.

Tests for Motor Effects of Facial Nerve

1. The subject is asked to raise the eyebrows. The furrows on the forehead are noted.
2. The subject is asked to shut his eyes as tightly as he can. An attempt to open the closed eyes against resistance is made.
3. The subject is asked to whistle. This is impossible in facial palsy.
4. The subject is asked to smile or show his upper teeth. In paralysis, the angle of the mouth in drawn to the healthy side.
5. He is asked to blow his cheeks and an attempt is made to deflate it by tapping on it with a finger. Air escapes more easily on the paralysed side.

Features of Facial Nerve Palsy (Motor Effects)

Affected Side Shows

1. Loss of expression.
2. Nasolabial fold would be less pronounced.
3. Furrows of the forehead would be smoothened.
4. Eye would be more widely open than on the normal side

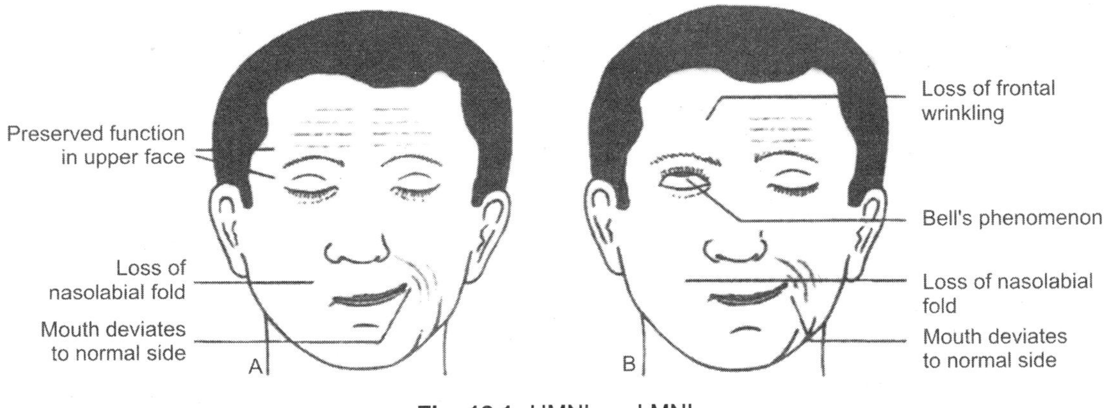

Fig. 13.1: UMNL vs LMNL

Student's Notes

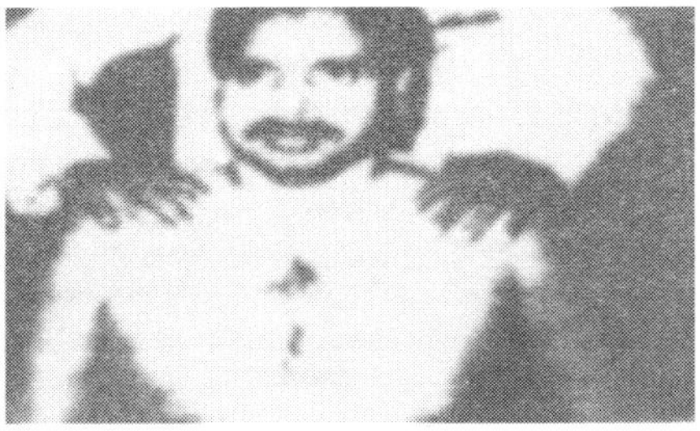

Fig. 13.2: Testing the spinal accessory nerve

5. Mouth is drawn towards the normal side when the patient smiles.
6. Unable to whistle.
7. Food collects between the teeth and cheek.
8. Saliva escapes from the affected angle of the mouth.

Supranuclear Facial Paralysis

Lower part of the face chiefly affected since the upper part is bilaterally innervated. Taste is not affected.

Infranuclear Facial Paralysis (lesion of the nucleus of facial nerve)

Both upper and lower part equally involved. Since it is a lower motor neuron lesion, the facial muscles show atrophy at a later date (Bell's palsy). Chorda tympani branch affected, if the lesion is in the facial canal—loss of taste sensation in the anterior two-thirds of the tongue. If the stapedius is paralysed, the sound on the affected side may be—unusually loud (hyperacusis).

VII. VESTIBULOCOCHLEAR NERVE

It contains two sets of fibres: (a) Auditory and (b) vestibular.

Auditory Pathway

From cochlear ganglion, the fibres enter the brainstem and distribute in the dorsal and ventral cochlear nuclei. The secondary auditory tracts, after partial decussation, terminate in the inferior colliculi and medial geniculate bodies. The fibres then pass via the internal capsule to the centre for hearing in the auditory cortex in the temporal lobe.

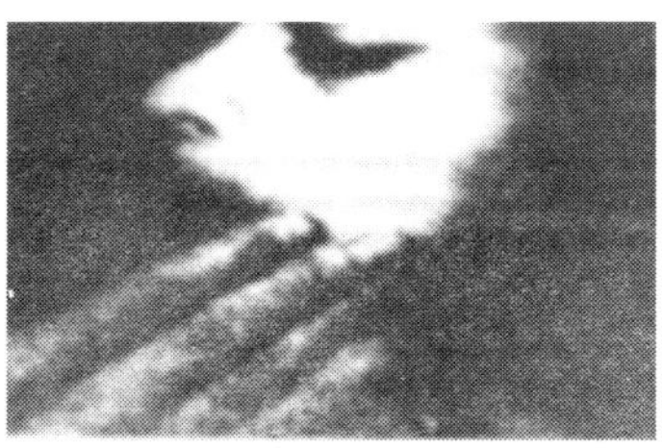

Fig. 13.3: Testing the hypoglossal nerve

Vestibular Pathway

From the semicircular canals and labyrinth (sense of equilibrium and balance) and through the vestibular ganglion, the fibers terminate in the vestibular nuclei of pons and medulla.

This has got close connections with the cerebellum and temporal lobe of cerebral cortex.

Tests for Hearing

1. The subject's capacity for hearing conversational and whispered voice is to be found.
2. *Tuning fork tests:* A tuning fork with a frequency of 256 or 128 Hz is used.
   a. *Rinne's test:* The prongs of the tuning fork is struck and the base is kept on the mastoid process. Once the sound is no more heard, the tuning fork is held near the pinna of the ear to perceive the sound once again. In a normal person, air conduction is better than bone conduction (Rinne's positive). In sensorineural deafness (lesion of cochlear branch of VIII nerve), Rinne is positive as long as the deafness is partial. In conductive deafness, Rinne is negative.
   b. *Weber's test:* The vibrating tuning fork is kept in the vertex of the forehead. In a normal person, the sound would be heard well on both sides. In conductive deafness (middle ear deafness), sound is perceived better in the affected ear. In sensorineural deafness, the sound is louder in the better hearing ear.
   c. *Schwabach test:* In this test, the bone conduction is compared to that of the examiner. The prongs of the tuning fork is struck and the base is kept on the mastoid process. Once the subject is unable to hear, the base is brought to the examiner's mastoid process to assess, if the sound is still heard or not.
3. *Audiometry tests:* Used to assess the degree of hearing loss and the likely site of pathology in the auditory pathway.
   a. Pure tone audiometry.
   b. Speech audiometry.

Abnormal Auditory Sensations

1. Tinnitus.
2. Hyperacusis—even slight sounds are heard with painful intensity (due to paralysis of stapedius muscle).

Vestibular Nerve Tests

Caloric test: Water is added 7°C above and below the normal body temperature (37°C) with the head postioned at 30° and nystagmus is looked for.

Student's Notes

IX. GLOSSOPHARYNGEAL NERVE

Anatomy

Receives sensory sensations from the posterior one-third of the tongue and the mucous membranes of the pharynx. It also receives taste sensation from posterior one-third of the tongue.

It also innervates the middle pharyngeal sphincter and stylopharyngeus muscle.

Tests

a. The taste sensation in posterior one-third of the tongue is examined.
b. The back of the pharynx is tickled (pharyngeal reflex). Reflex contraction of pharyngal muscles results.

X. VAGUS NERVE

Anatomy

It gives motor innervation for soft palate (except tensor palati) pharynx and larynx.

Sensory and motor supply for respiratory passage and heart. Parasympathetic supply to the abdominal viscera.

Tests

1. The subject is asked whether there is any regurgitation of fluids through the nose while swallowing. This occurs in total paralysis of soft palate.
2. The subject is asked to say high pitched word like 'egg' and 'rub' which requires complete closure of nasopharynx. In paralysis of vagus, 'egg' is pronounced as 'eng' and 'rub' as 'rum'.
3. The subject is asked to say 'Ah'. In bilateral paralysis, the soft palate remains motionless. In unilateral paralysis, the affected side remains motionless.
4. Visceral reflex—oculocardiac and carotid sinus reflex (not done in class).

XI. ACCESSORY NERVE

Anatomy

It is purely motor nerve. It has got a cranial and a spinal origin. It innervates some muscles of pharynx and larynx as well as sternomastoid and trapezius.

1. *Test for trapezius:* The subject is asked to shrug his shoulder against resistance.
2. *Test for sternomastoid:* The subject is asked to rotate his chin against resistance.

XII. HYPOGLOSSAL NERVE

Anatomy

It is a motor nerve, it supplies the tongue and the depressors of the hyoid.

Test

1. The subject is asked to protrude the tongue. In unilateral lesion, the tongue would deviate to the paralysed side.
2. The subject is asked to move the tongue from side to side and to lick each lip with it. Observe whether this can be done freely. Strength may also be assessed by pressing against the tongue with a finger as the subject protrudes it into each cheek.
3. Fasciculation and wasting of the muscle is also looked for. Fasciculation is assessed with the tongue relaxed in the mouth not when protruded. Wasting indicates lower motor neuron paralysis.

QUESTIONS

1. Differentiate between, lower motor and upper motor neuron lesions of the facial nerve.
2. What are the muscles of facial expressions?
3. What is the receptor for taste sensation?
4. Trace the pathway for taste sensation from the tongue.
5. What is aguesia and paraguesia? Give examples.
6. What are the bed side tests for hearing?
7. What is hyperacusis? When does a person get hyperacusis?
8. What is the principle behind tuning fork test?
9. What is the receptor for hearing and centre for hearing?
10. Mention 2 types of deafness and list the tests to differentiate these types.
11. What is the afferent nerve and efferent nerve for palatal reflex?
12. What is gag reflex?
13. What is nystagmus? What are its components? Name some conditions which cause nystagmus.
14. Name the visceral reflex for the X nerve.
15. What are the muscles supplied by the XI nerve?
16. Name some tests for the vestibular division of VIII nerve.
17. Name the intrinsic muscles of the tongue?
18. Which side is the tongue deviated if the XII nerve is paralysed on the left side'?
19. What is Bell's palsy?
20. How will you treat Bell's palsy?
21. What are the tests for motor division of facial nerve?
22. Why dose the upper part of the face not affected in supranuclear lesion of the VIIth nerve?
23. What is vertigo?
24. What is fasciculation? How will you test it ?
25. What are the effects of paralysis of IX cranial nerve?

Student's Notes

26. What are the two types of nerves which supply the tongue and mention their areas.
27. What are primary taste sensation and where are they found.
28. What is ptosis? In which type of facial nerve palsy it is found?
29. What is common cause of loss of hearing?
30. What is dysarthria?

EXAMINATION OF CRANIAL NERVES VII TO XII

Name: .... Age: ....

Sex: .... Occupation: ....

General Examination

Higher function

VII Nerve

Sensory examination	*Right*	*Left*
Taste sensation in anterior two-thirds		
Sweet (sugar)		
Salt (salt)		
Sour (vinegar)		
Bitter (quinine)		

Motor examination	*Right*	*Left*
Raise eyebrows		
Shut eyes tightly		
Whistle		
Smile (nasolabial fold)		
Show upper teeth (angle of mouth)		

VIII Vestibulocochlear Nerve

Bed side test	*Right*	*Left*
Whispering		
Watch test		
Rubbing of fingers		

Tuning fork test	*Right*	*Left*
Rinne's test		
Weber's test		
Schwabach test		

IX Glossopharyngeal Nerve	*Right*	*Left*
Taste sensation in posterior one-third of tongue		
Sweet		
Salt		
Bitter		
Sour		
Pharyngeal reflex		

Student's Notes

X Vagus	Right	Left
1. Regurgitation of fluids		
2. Say high pitched sound		
3. Say"Ah"		
4. Pharyngeal reflex		

XI Accessory Nerve	Right	Left
1. Shrug shoulder against resistance		
2. Rotate chin against resistance		

XII Hypoglossal Nerves	Right	Left
1. Protrude the tongue		
2. Move tongue from side to side		
3. Fasciculation		
4. Wasting		

Inference:

Experiment 14: Perimetry

Aim

To chart the uniocular visual field of a given subject using Lister's perimeter.

Definition of Visual Field

The field of vision is defined as the sum of the objects that form images on the retina when the eye is fixed at a particular point. Various methods are available for measuring the field of vision.

Perimetry

The instrument used for accurate charting of the field of vision is called a perimeter. It consists of metal arc graduated in degrees. The metal arc is either a quardrant or semicircle of a circle. The concavity of the arc faces the subject. A holder sliding in the arc carries a test object which can be glided along the length of the arc. The arc is pivoted at the centre and can be rotated through various angle. For plotting the field of vision, test object of different colours and sizes can be used. The subject is asked to rest his chin on one of the two chin rests. When the field of the right eye is to be plotted, the subject rests his chin on the left chin rest. This brings his eye in line with the fixation point.

Before mapping the field of vision, the perimetry chart is studied. The lines through the centre of the circle denotes the various meridian in degrees. Each concentric circle around the centre denote points of equal visual acuity called isopters and are marked in degrees from the central fixation point. The perimter is used to chart the visual field between the periphery and the 30 isopter circle. The metal arc is adjusted in one meridian and the object is then brought gradually from the periphery (90°) towards the centre (fixation point). Keeping the eye on the central fixation point, the subject is asked to point at which he just sees the object. This reading in degrees on the arc is marked on the chart for that articular meridian. In this way, the procedure is repeated at every 15° intervals till the field of vision is plotted in four quadrant. Care is to be taken to mark the blind spot along the horizontal meridian in the temporal quadrant.

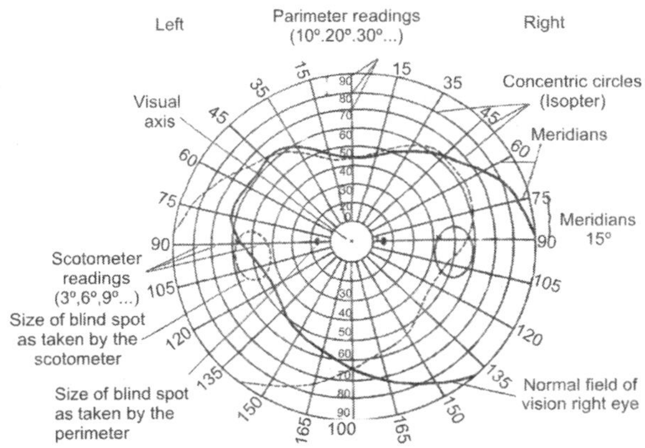

Fig. 14.2: Perimetric chart

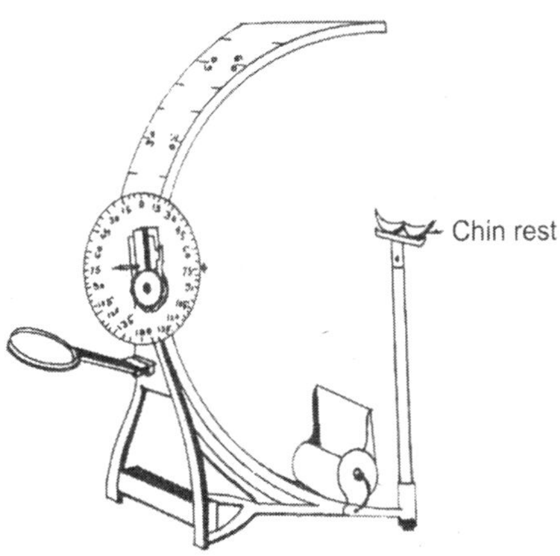

Fig. 14.1: Perimeter

QUESTIONS

1. Give the medial, lateral, superior and inferior extent of the field of vision. Explain the differences in the various extents.
2. Draw a diagram to show the possible lesions in the optic tract and the resultiant defects in the field of vision.
3. Mention the precautions for performing perimetry.
4. Mention the factors affecting the field of vision.
5. What is blind spot?
6. What is tubular vision?
7. What happens when there is damage to optic chiasma centrally and peripherally?
8. What is optic radiation?
9. What are the uses of perimetry?
10. What is binocular vision?
11. What is bitemporal hemianopia and its cause?
12. What is binasal hemianopia and its cause?
13. What is homonymous hemianopia?
14. What is stereoscopic vision ?
15. What is scotoma?
16. Name any other method of determining the field of vision?

Student's Notes

Experiment 15: Cerebellar Function Tests

Cerebellum plays a major role in co-ordination of rapid muscular activities and helps to sequence the motor activities and also monitors and makes corrective adjustments in the body motor activities as they are performed.

In cerebellar dysfunction, the movements ordinarily overshoot their intended mark.

This effect is called dysmetria and it results in inco-ordinated movements that are called ataxia.

Tests for ataxia and dysmetria:

1. *Past pointing:* When the subject attempts to touch an object with a finger, it results in overshooting to one side or the other.
2. *Finger–nose test:* The subject is asked to touch his nose with one index finger and then with the other with eyes open.
3. *Finger–finger–nose test:* The subject is asked to touch his nose first and then the examiner's forefinger with his index finger.
4. *Counting:* The subject is asked to touch each finger in turn with the thumbs rapidly.

Dysdiadochokinesia is the inability to perform rapidly alternating opposite movements. The subject is asked to flex the elbow to a right angle and then alternately supinate and pronate the forearm as rapidly as possible.

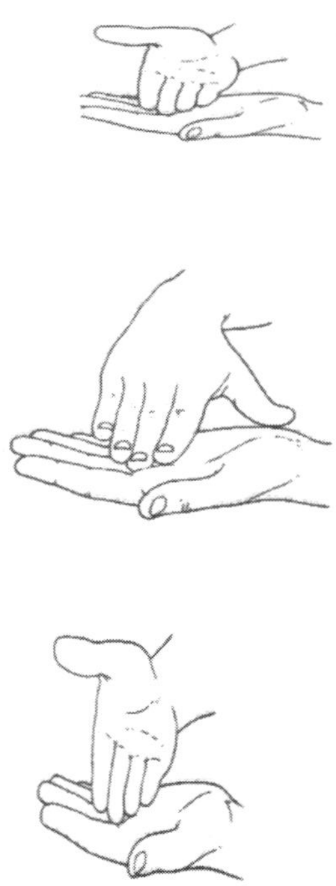

Fig. 15.1: Looking for dysdiadochokinesis

Other tests for co-ordination:

1. Everyday movements like dressing or undressing, handling a book, picking up pins, threading a needle are observed.
2. *Heel-shin ankle test:* In cerebellar ataxia, a characteristic irregular side to side series of errors in the speed and direction of movement occurs. The test should be performed with eyes open.
3. The subject is asked to draw a large circle in the air with the toe and put a dot in the centre. In cerebellar ataxia, it is squared off irregularly.
4. The subject is asked to walk along a straight line.

Dysarthria is the defective articulation of speech. The subject speaks slowly and deliberately syllable by syllable as in scanning a line. EGG is pronounced as ENG. This staccato speech rhythm is characteristic of severe cerebellar dysarthria. Minor cerebellar dysarthria causes slowing and slurring of speech.

Intentional Tremor or Action Tremor

When a person with cerebellar dysfunction performs a voluntary act, the movements oscillate, especially when they approach the intended mark. The subject is asked to lift an object such as a glass of water, and the presence of tremors is looked for.

Nystagmus

Cerebellar nystagmus is a tremor of the eyeballs that occurs usually when one attempts to fix the eyes on a scene to one side of the head.

Hypotonia in cerebellar disease, there is decreased tone of the peripheral body musculature on the side of the lesion.

Rebound Phenomenon

The subject is asked to flex the forearm against resistance. If the resistance is suddenly withdrawn, the patient cannot break the movement of the limb and the forearm sways backward in the wide arc. This is because in cerebellar diseases, the patient is unable to stop movement promptly.

Decompensation of movement: In performing a complex action involving more than one joint, e.g. touching the back of the head with the finger, it is not done smoothly as one movement is split into its component parts.

Student's Notes

Pendular knee jerk: After eliciting patellar tendon reflex, the limb will swing back and forth, like a pendulum a few times, because of hypotonia.

Gait: Reeling or drunken gait occurs in cerebellar ataxia. Patients with this gait disorder walk on a broad base with the feet placed widely apart and irregularly.

QUESTIONS

1. Name the organs responsible for equilibrium.
2. Name the vestibular apparatus?
3. Name the three types of cerebellum phylogenetically.
4. Name the nucleus of the cerebellum.
5. What is dysdiadochokinesis? Examples?
6. What is intentional tremor and resting tremor?
7. What is tetany?
8. What is Rhomberg sign?
9. Name the two ascending spino-cerebellar test?
10. What is dysmetria?
11. What is nystagmus?
12. What is tinnitus?
13. What is the receptor in the semicircular canals and otolith organs?
14. How is the cerebellum connected to the brainstem?
15. Which nucleus of the cerebellum is concerned with coordination? Name the tract connecting this to the cortex.
16. Mention some abnormal gaits.

CEREBELLAR FUNCTION TEST

Name: .... Age: ....

Sex: .... Occupation: ....

Upper Limb

Tone - both sides

	EYES OPEN		EYES CLOSED	
	Right	*Left*	*Right*	*Left*
Finger–nose test				
Finger–finger–nose test				
Counting of fingers				
Dysdiadochokinesia				
Rebound phenomenon				
Threading a needle				

Lower Limb

Gait

Tone - Both sides

Knee-jerk - Both sides

Walk along a straight line

Tandem walk

	EYES OPEN		EYES CLOSED	
	Right	*Left*	*Right*	*Left*
Knee heel test				
Draw a circle and put a dot in centre				

Romberg's sign

Others

Speech

Nystagmus

Inference:

Student's Notes

1

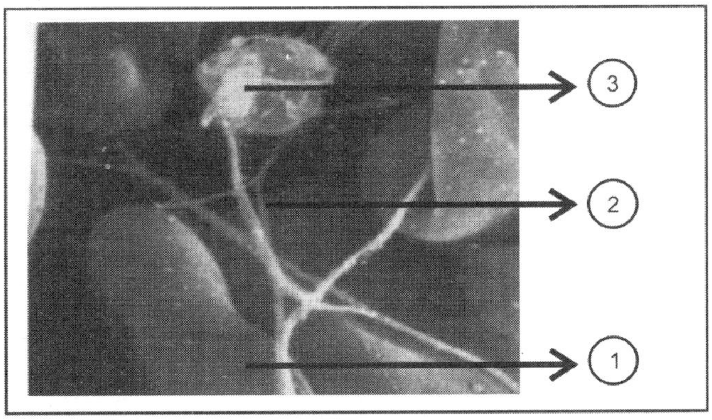

1. Identify the structures 1, 2, 3.
2. What is the function of 3?
3. Name the IV, VIII, X clotting factor?
4. What is the difference between extrinsic and intrinsic coagulation?

COMMENT/ANSWER

Blood Clotting

1. 1-RBC, 2-Fibrin threads, 3-Platelets
2. It plays a vital role in all steps of hemostasis
   i. Vasospasm – 5HT.
   ii. Platelet plug formation—thromboxine A_2.
   iii. Fibrin thread formation.
   iv. Clot retraction (actin filaments).
   v. Fibrinolysis
   vi. Production of platelet derived growth factor (PDGF).
3. IV – Calcium
   VIII – Antihemophilic factor A
   X – Stuart prower factor.
4. **Intrinsic pathway**
   i. Initiated on damage to vessel wall and exposure to collagen.
   ii. Initiated with factor XII.
   iii. Platelets are required.
   iv. Slow process—takes few minutes.
   v. Clotting time and thromboplastin

   Extrinsic pathway
   i. Initiated on damage to tissue.
   ii. Initiated with factor III.
   iii. Platelets are not required.
   iv. Fast process–takes few seconds.
   v. Prothrombin time is a test for generation test are used pathways.

2

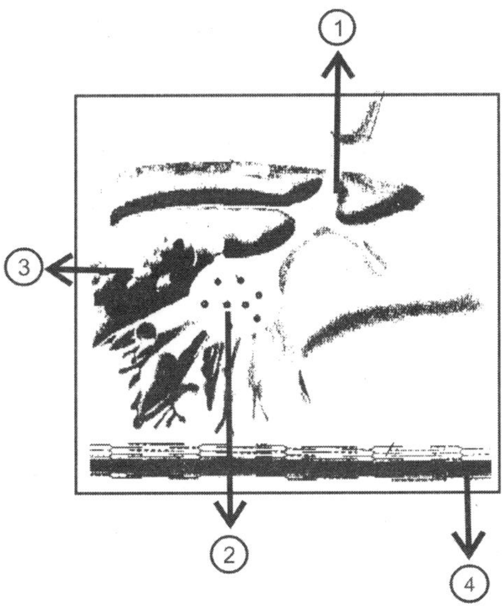

1. Identify 1, 2, 3, 4.
2. What is the neurotransmitter released here?
3. Which receptor do they act?
4. Name the potential developed by this junction .
5. Name any two neuromuscular blockers .

COMMENT/ANSWER

Neuromuscular Junction

1. 1–Nerve terminal, 2–Motor end plate, 3–Vesicle, 4–Muscle fibre.
2. Acetyl choline
3. Nicotinic receptor
4. End plate potential
5. Tubocurarine and succinyl choline

3

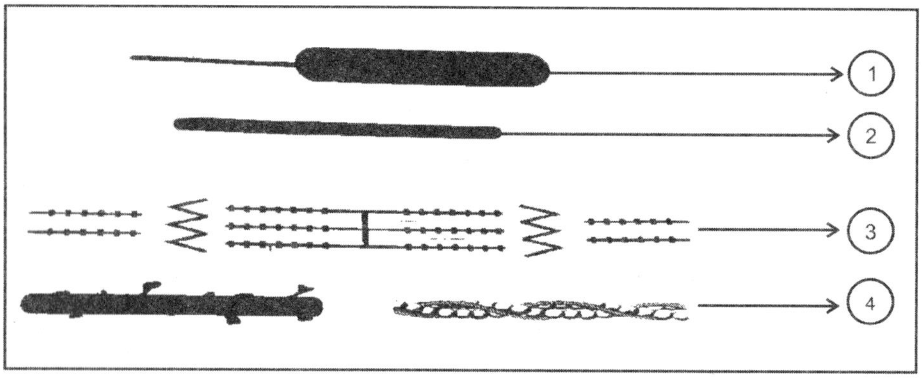

1. Identify 1, 2, 3, 4, 5.
2. What is the function of 4 and 5 ?
3. What does it contain ?

COMMENT/ANSWER

Skeletal Muscle Fibre

1. 1–Muscle fibre, 2–Myofibril, 3–Myofilament, 4–Actin filament, 5–Myosin filament
2. Actin and myosin filaments slide on each other causing muscle contraction by sliding filament theory.
3. 4 contains G-actin molecule forming f-actin polymer(double helix), tropomyosin, troponin. 5 contains myosin molecules having 2 heavy chains and 4 light chains (head, hinge and rod).

4

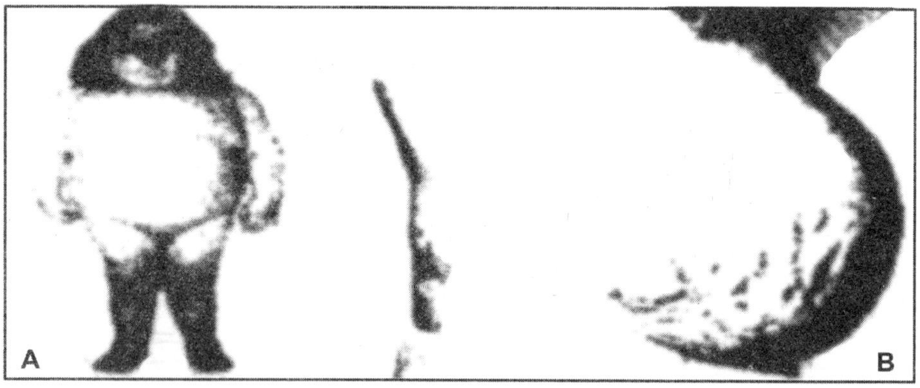

1. Identify the pictures A and B. What is the cause for the pathophysiology in picture B?
2. Explain the other clinical features of this condition.
3. What is the commonest cause for this condition?

COMMENT/ANSWER

Cushing's Syndrome

1. A is Cushing's syndrome, B is purple striae on the skin and the abdomen. The cause of this pathophysiology in B is rupture of the subcutaneous tissue due to catabolic effect of cortisol.
2. Moon face, buffalo hump, truncal obesity, thin limbs, muscular wasting, hirsutism.
3. Iatrogenic or doctor induced–over dosage of steroids. Adrenal hyperplasia or tumour.

5

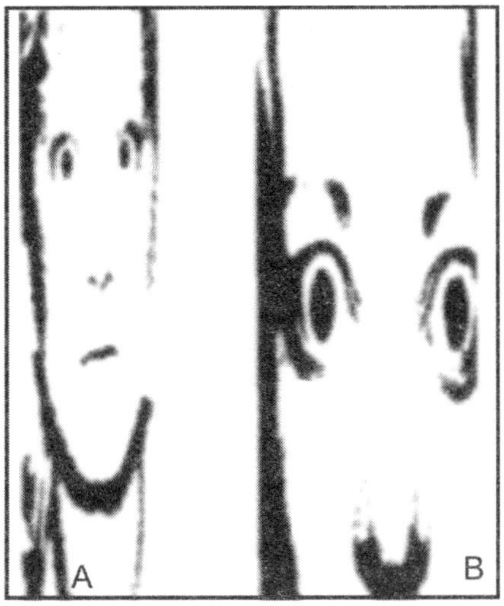

1. Identify the pictures A and B.
2. What is the cause for this condition?
3. What will be the salient clinical features of this subject?

COMMENT/ANSWER

Exophthalmos

1. A and B are cases of hyperthyroidism with classic features of exophthalmos.
2. Increased T3 and T4 levels in the blood. It is considered to be an autoimmune disease.
3. Increased BMR, increased sweating, fine tremors, nervousness and tachycardia with atrial fibrillation.

6

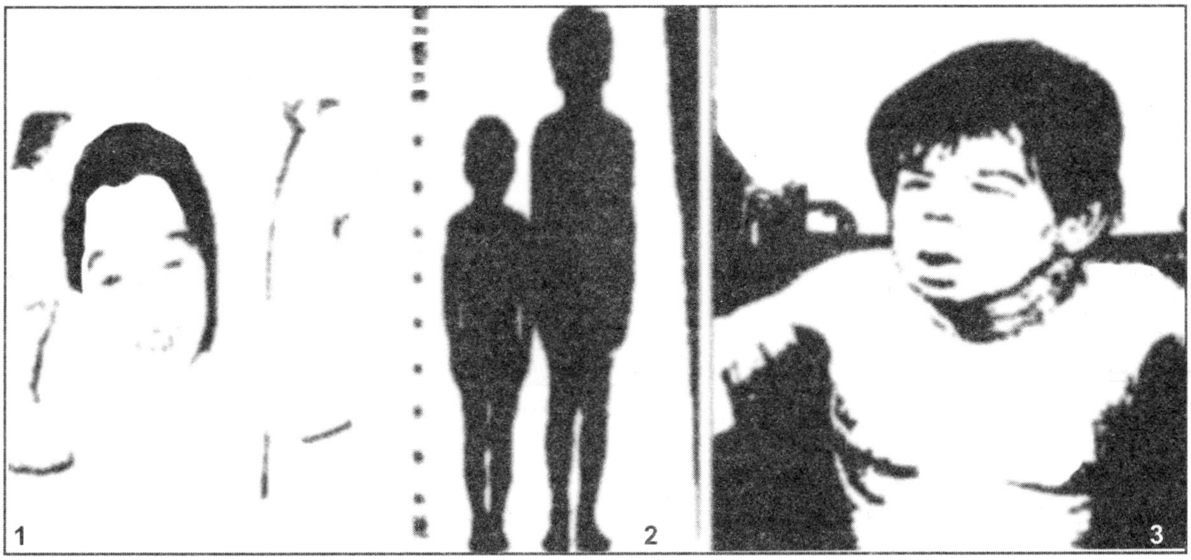

1. Identify 1, 2, 3. What is its cause?
2. What is the neurological manifestation of this child and why?
3. What other clinical features are seen in this subject?

COMMENT/ANSWER

Cretinism of Newborn

1. 1–Cretinism of newborn, 2–Stunted growth, dry scaly skin, 3–Classical features of cretinism
2. Mental retardation due to non-myelination of central nervous system.
3. Loss of appetite, increased BMR, intolerance to heat, idiotic look and behaviour.

7

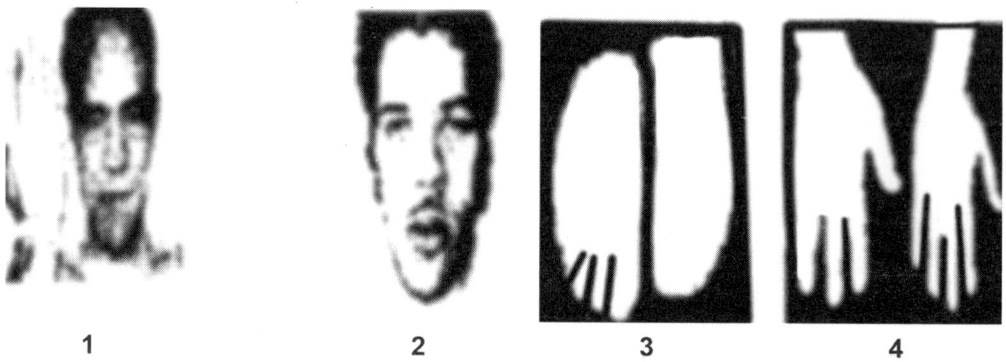

1. Identify the pictures in 1, 2, 3, 4.
2. What other clinical features are seen in this condition?
3. How can you treat this condition?

COMMENT/ANSWER

Myxoedema

1. Features of hypothyroidism in adult–myxoedema. 1 and 2 myxematous face with lethargic tired look. 3 Lid lag in myxoedema, 4 non-pitting type of oedema in lower limb.
2. Hoarse voice, intolerance to cold, bradycardia, constipation, loss of appetite, tiredness, decreased BMR.
3. Administration of levothyroxine tablets regularly.

8

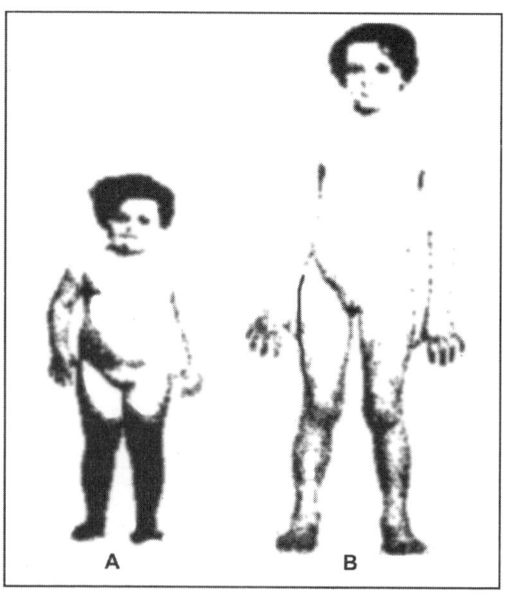

1. Identify A and B. Which is the abnormal person here?
2. Give your reasons.
3. What are the other different varieties of this disorder?

COMMENT/ANSWER

Dwarfism

1. A–Dwarf, B–Normal child of same age. In this picture, A is abnormal.
2. Decreased growth hormone before the fusion of epiphysis.
3. A. Sexual atellotic dwarfism, B. Lorain dwarfism (pigmies dwarfism), C. Lorain-Levy dwarfism

9

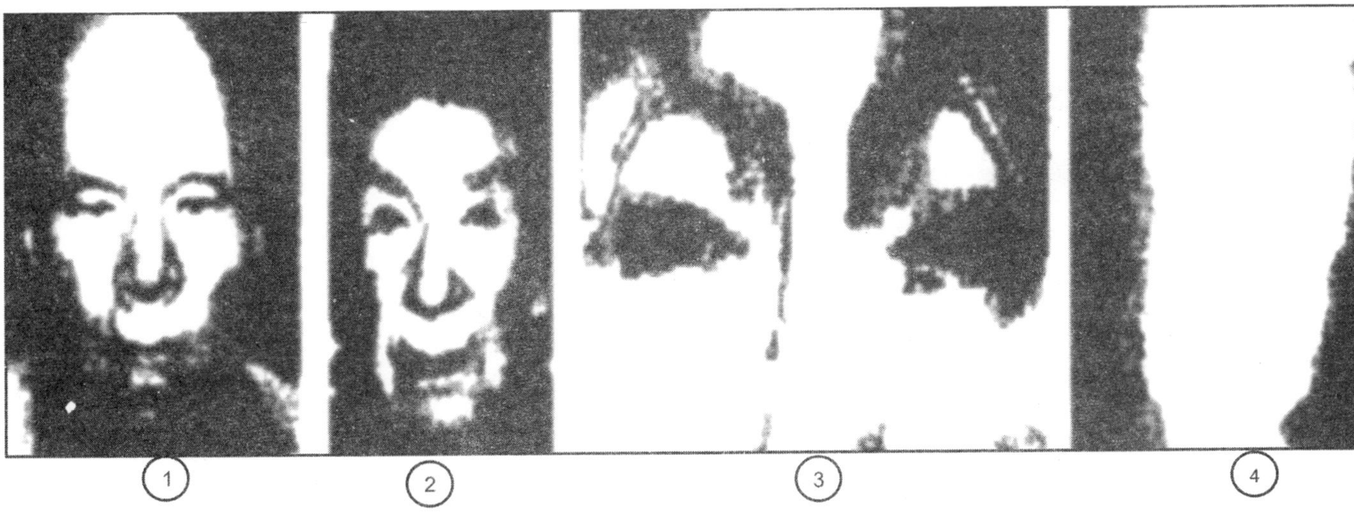

1. Identify the pictures in 1, 2, 3, 4.
2. What other clinical features are seen in this condition?
3. How can you treat this condition?

COMMENT/ANSWER

Myxoedema

1. Features of hypothyroidism in adult–myxoedema. 1 and 2 Myxedematous face with lethargic tired look, 3 Lid lag in myxoedema, 4 Non-pitting type of oedema in lower limb.
2. Hoarse voice, intolerance to cold, bradycardia, constipation, loss of appetite, tiredness, decreased BMR.
3. Administration of levothyroxine tablets regularly.

10

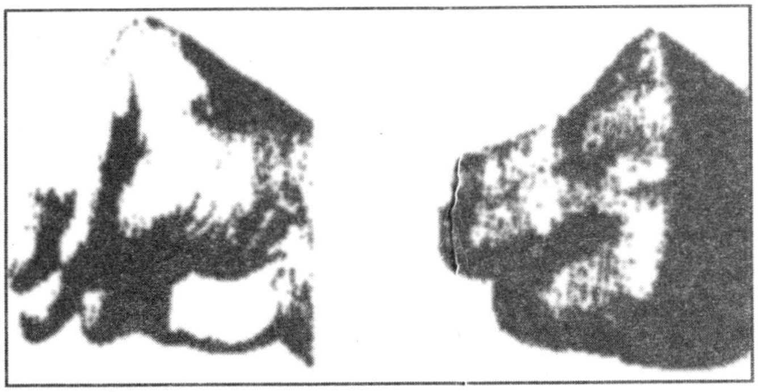

1. Identify this condition and its cause.
2. What are the other signs seen in this disorder?
3. Name the hormones which control the ion related to this disorder.

COMMENT/ANSWER

Carpopedal Spasm

1. Carpopedal spasm/tetany/Accoucher's/obstetrician hand in hypoparathyroidism. Cause—when plasma calcium is decreased to 7.5 mg%.
2. Trousseau's sign. Chevostek's sign–due to hyperexcitability of nerve.
3. Parathormone, calcitonin and vitamin D.

11

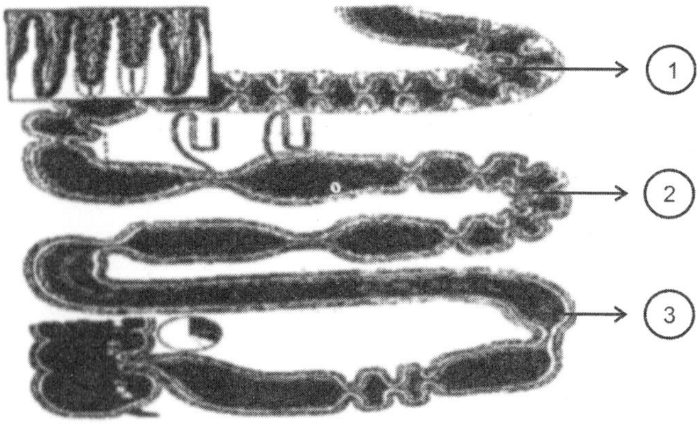

1. Identify the arrows 1 , 2 and 3.
2. What is the function of each of these movements?
3. Which nerve plexus is responsible?

COMMENT/ANSWER

Intestinal Movements

1. i. Segmental rhythmic contractions.
   ii. Peristalsis or propulsive contractions.
   iii. Peristaltic rush.
2. Function of these movements are:
   i. Grinding or mixing of food with digestive juices and absorption .
   ii. Movement from oral to aboral end.
   iii. To evacuate the contents that irritate the alimentary tract.
3. Myentric plexus.

12

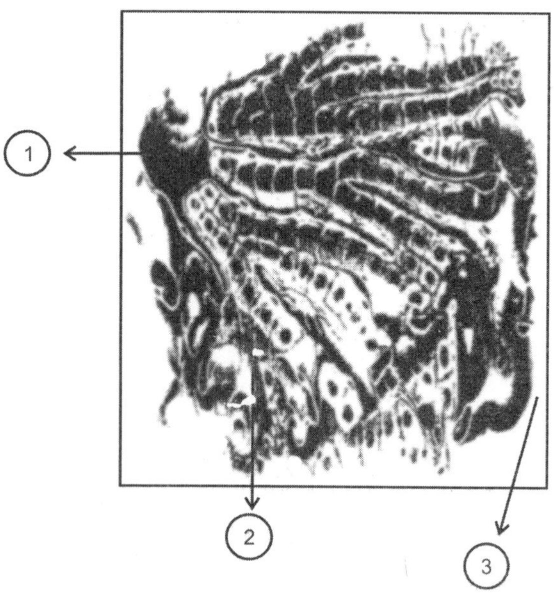

1. Identify 1, 2, 3.
2. What is the function of structure 2?
3. What is enterohepatic circulation?

COMMENT/ANSWER

Biliary System–Hepatocytes

1. i. Central vein
   ii. Hepatocyte
   iii. Portal vein
2. Secretion of bile.
3. Enterohepatic circulation–Bile salts that are secreted in bile again enter the liver through the portal circulation. This is called enterohepatic circulation.

13

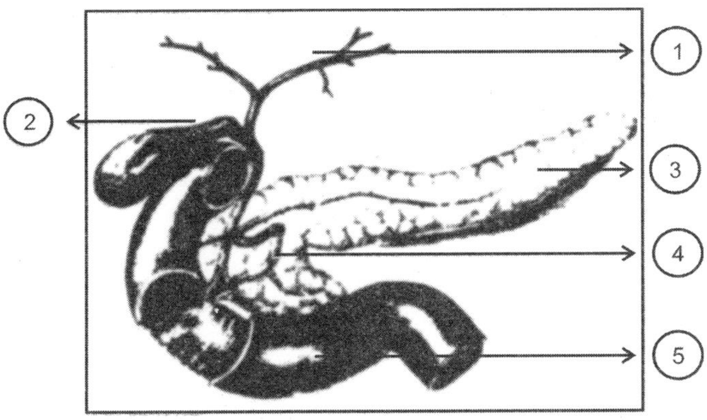

1. Identify 1, 2, 3, 4, 5.
2. What is the function of the structure 2 and 3?
3. Name the bile salts. What are choleretics and cholegogues?

COMMENT/ANSWER

Gallbladder with Biliary Duct, Pancreas and Duodenum

1. 1–Bile duct, 2–Gallbladder, 3–Pancreas, 4–Ampulla of vater, 5–3rd part of duodenum
2. Function of 2: Concentration of bile, Function of 3: Secretion of pancreatic juice, exocrine—enzymes, endocrine—insulin, glucagon.
3. Bile salts–Na and K salts of Tauro and glycocholates of bile acid. Choleretics–substances that increase the formation of bile.
   Bile salt, ACh, cholegogues–substances that make contraction of gallbladder–CCK, gastrin, ACh.

14

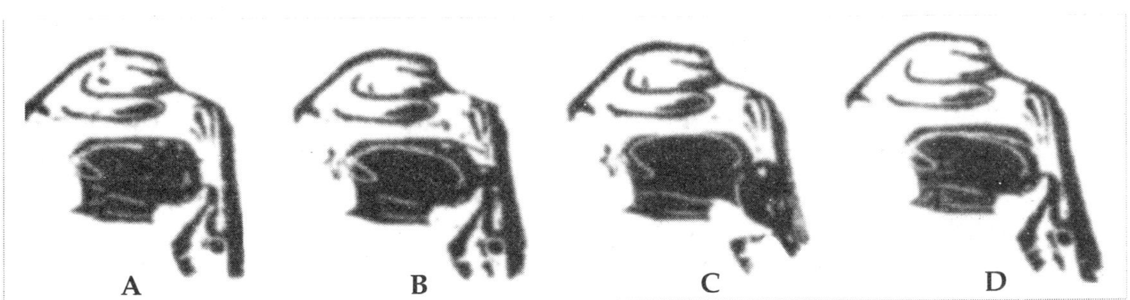

1. Identify the structures A, B, C, D.
2. Why food does not enter the larynx?
3. Where is the deglutition centre situated?
4. Which stage is the voluntary stage ?

COMMENT/ANSWER

Stages of Deglutition

1. Various stages of deglutition: A. Oral stage, B. Oral stage, C. Pharyngeal stage, D. Esophageal stage.
2. Temporary cessation of breathing (apnoea), approximation of vocal cords and closure of the laryngeal inlet by the epiglottis.
3. In the medulla.
4. Oral stage

15

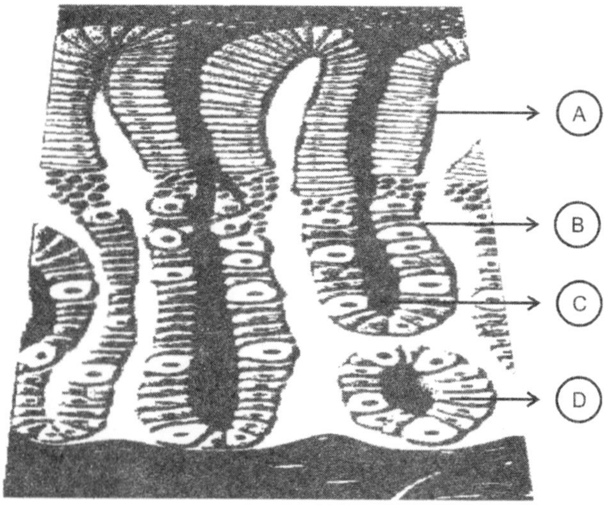

1. Identify A, B, C and D.
2. Name the substances secreted by A, B, C and D?

COMMENT/ANSWER

Gastric Glands

1. a. Surface mucous cells
   b. Mucous like cells
   c. Parietal cells
   d. Chief cells
   e. G cells
2. a. Secretes insoluble mucous
   b. Secretes soluble mucous
   c. HCl and intrinsic factor
   d. Pepsinogen
   e. Gastrin

16

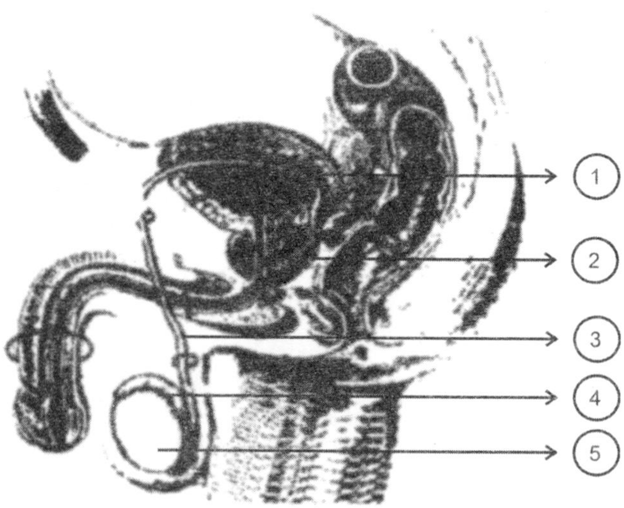

1. Identify the structures in the number 1 to 5.
2. What is the function of each of thess structures?

COMMENT/ANSWER

Male Reproductive System

1. 1–Seminal vesicle, 2–Prostate gland, 3–Vas deferens, 4–Epididymis, 5–Testis
2. Function of each:
   1. Contains prostaglandins and increase motility of sperm.
   2. Secrete spermin which further increases the motility of sperms and capacitation.
   3. Transport semen
   4. Maturation of sperms
   5. Production of sperms and hormones like testosterone, inhibin.

17

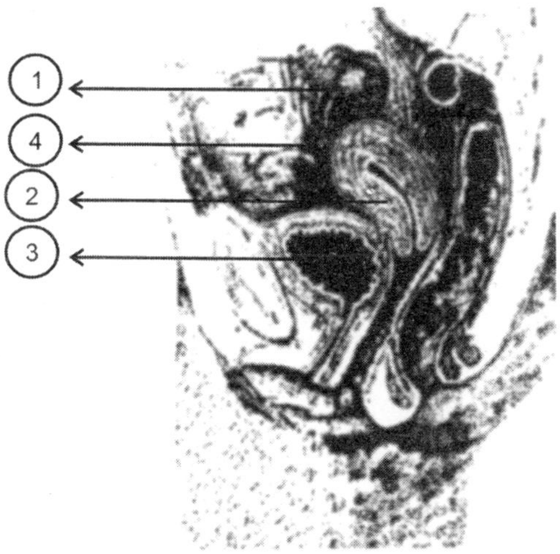

1. Identify the structures in the number 1 to 4.
2. What is the function of each of these structures?

COMMENT/ANSWER

Female Reproductive System

1. 1–Ovary, 2–Uterus, 3–Urinary bladder, 4–Fallopian tube.
2. Function of each:
   1. Production of ovum or egg.
   2. Implantation and growth of fetus and placenta.
   3. Collect and store the urine and micturition reflex.
   4. Transport the fertilized ova from the ovary to the uterus for implantation.

18

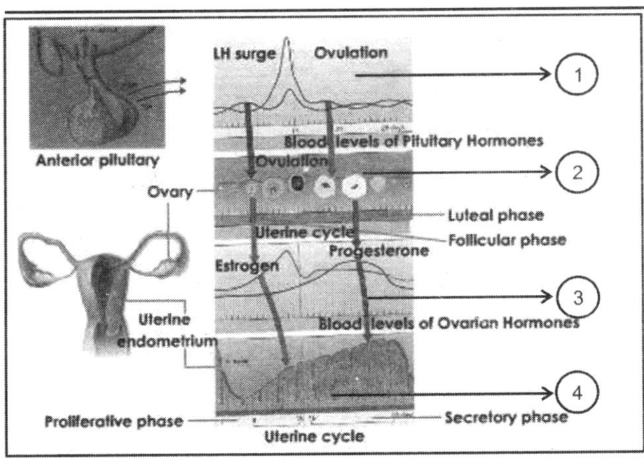

1. Identify the structures 1, 2, 3 and 4.
2. What are the various phases of this cycle?
3. Mention the hormones responsible for these changes.

COMMENT/ANSWER

Menstrual Cycle

1. These pictures show the events of:
   1. Gonadotrophic hormone cycles—connected with normal menstrual cycle.
   2. Ovarian cycles—during normal female sexual cycle.
   3. Ovarian hormone cycles—during normal female sexual cycle.
   4. Endometrial changes—during normal female sexual cycle.
2. Follicular and luteal phases of the ovarian cycle. Proliferative and secretory phases of endometrial cycle.
3. FSH is important for the development of the ovarian follicles. LH controls:
   1. Ovulation–by LH surge.
   2. Development of corpus luteum.
   3. Maintains pregnancy.

   Oestrogen and progesterone maintain the follicular and secretory phases of menstrual cycle.

19

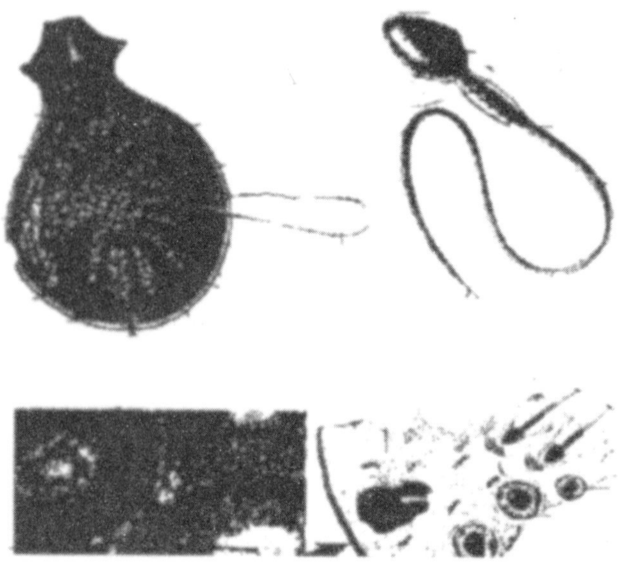

1. Identify the structures 1 to 3.
2. Enumerate the function of structure 3.

COMMENT/ANSWER

Spermiogenesis

1. 1–Testis, 2–Sperm, 3–Sertoli cells
2. Sertoli cells causes:
   a. Secretion of inhibin, androgen binding protein and Mullerian inhibiting substance.
   b. Spermiogenesis
   c. Responsible for providing nutrition and forming blood testis barrier.

20

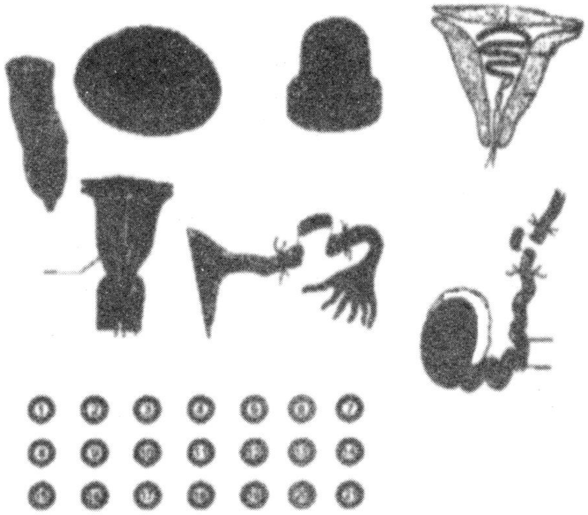

1. Identify the pictures 1 to 8.
2. Which is the best method and why?

COMMENT/ANSWER

Contraceptive Methods

1. 1–Condom, 2–Diaphragm, 3–Cervical cap, 4–Lippes' loop, 5–Copper-T, 6–Tubectomy, 7–Vasectomy, 8–Contraceptive pills
2. Hormonal pills is the best method because the success rate of contraception is high and it has least complications and it is also reversible.

21

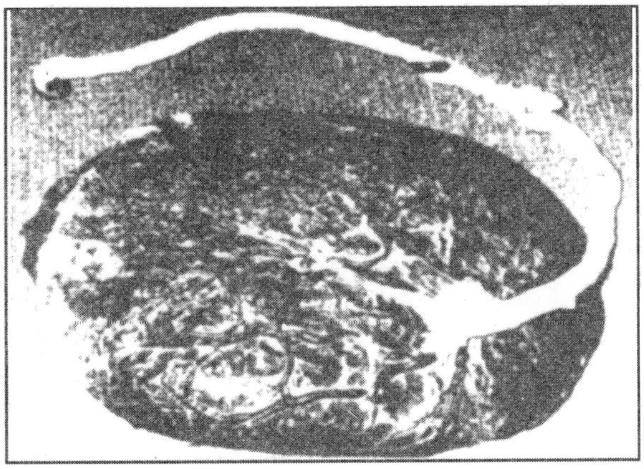

1. Identify the structure.
2. Name the hormones produced by this structure.
3. What is fetoplacental unit?

COMMENT/ANSWER

Placenta with Umbilical Cord

1. Placenta with umbilical cord.
2. HCG, estrogen, progesterone and relaxin.
3. Placenta uses the maternal and fetal segments to synthesize DHEA (dehydroepiandrosterone).

22

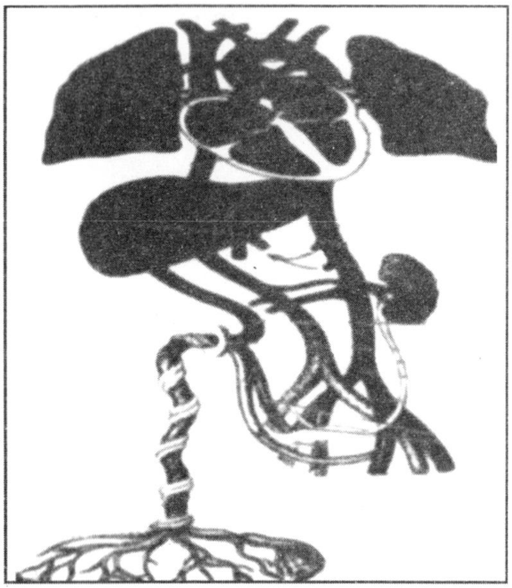

1. Identify this circulation.
2. Mention four peculiar features of this circulation.
3. What happens to this circulation after birth?

COMMENT/ANSWER

Fetal Circulation

1. This is fetal circulation.
2. i. Umbilical vein has blood which is 80% saturated with O_2.
   ii. A ductus venosus diverts some of the umbilical venous blood directly to IVC.
   iii. The resistance of collapsed lungs is higher than the pressure in the pulmonary artery. It is several mm Hg higher than aorta, so that most of the blood in the pulmonary artery passes through ductus arteriosus to aorta.
   iv. 55 % of fetal cardiac output goes through placenta.
3. At birth, the placental circulation is cut off and the peripheral resistance suddenly rises.The pressure in the aorta raises and till it exceeds than in the pulmonary artery. Hence infant becomes asphyxic. Therefore gasps for breath and the lungs expand. Pulmonary vascular resistance falls and pulmonary blood flow increases markedly. Ductus arteriosus closes. Foramen ovale closes.

23

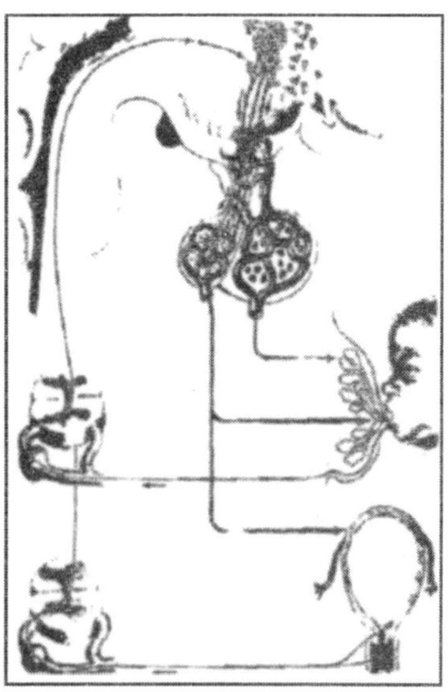

1. What is this reflex? What are the other names?
2. Name the nucleus which secretes the hormone. What is the other action of this hormone?

COMMENT/ANSWER

Sucking Reflex

1. Sucking reflex, neuroendocrine reflex—other names are milk ejection reflex, milk let down reflex.
2. Paraventricular nucleus and supraoptic nucleus of hypothalamus.
3. Parturition reflex (expulsion of foetus and placenta).

24

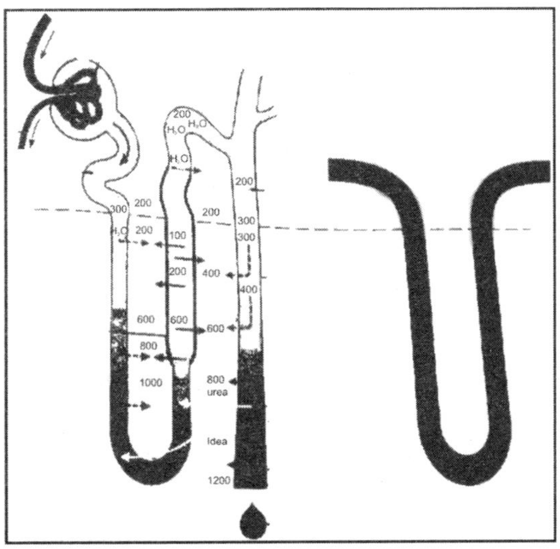

1. Identify the picture.
2. What mechanism is involved in two segments A and B?
3. Under what situation the, nephron will perform this mechanism?

COMMENT/ANSWER

Counter Current Mechanism

1. Loop of Henle and the vasa recta are involved in the concentration of urine.
2. A. Countercurrent multiplier system for forming a concentrated medullary gradient.

   B. Counter current exchange system for maintaining the medullary concentration gradient.
3. Dehydration due to excessive sweating, diarrhoea, vomiting and hemorrhage.

25

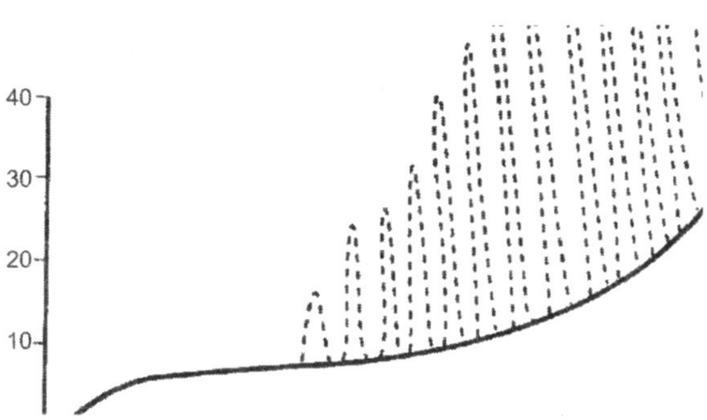

1. Identify the curve and describe the segments.
2. What is plasticity?
3. Name the law, this picture obeys?
4. Name three abnormal bladders

COMMENT/ANSWER

Cystometrogram

1. The curve is identified as a cystometrogram. The segments are 1a, 1b, and 2.
2. Plasticity is the property of the smooth muscle to behave as a viscous mass than a rigid structure. Detrussor muscle of the bladder is responsible for plasticity.
3. This picture obeys Laplace law.
4. The three abnormal bladders are:
   1. Automatic bladder, 2. Atonic bladder,
   3. Uninhibited neurogenic bladder.

26

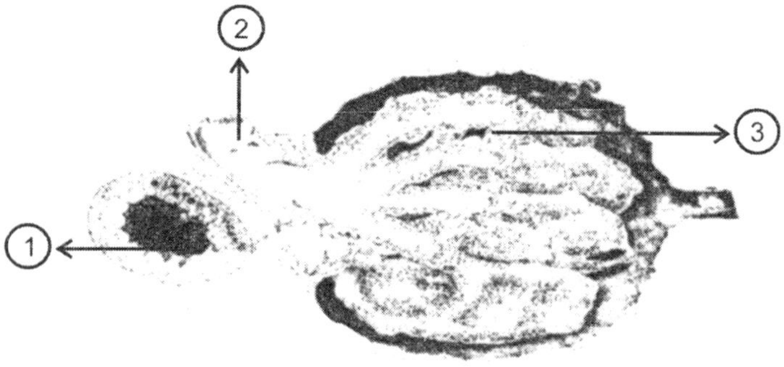

1. Identify the structures 1, 2, 3.
2. What is the function of each part?
3. What is tubuloglomerular feedback mechanism?

COMMENT/ANSWER

Juxtaglomerular Apparatus

1. 1–Macula densa, 2–Juxtaglomerular cells, 3–Extra glomerular mesangial cells.
2. The functions are:
   1. Macula densa is involved in the tubuloglomerular feedback mechanism, 2. J G cells secrete renin, 3. Extraglomerular mesangial cells—its function is not known.
3. The tubuloglomerular feedback is the interaction between the distal tubules and the glomerulus in maintaining the autoregulation in the kidney.

27

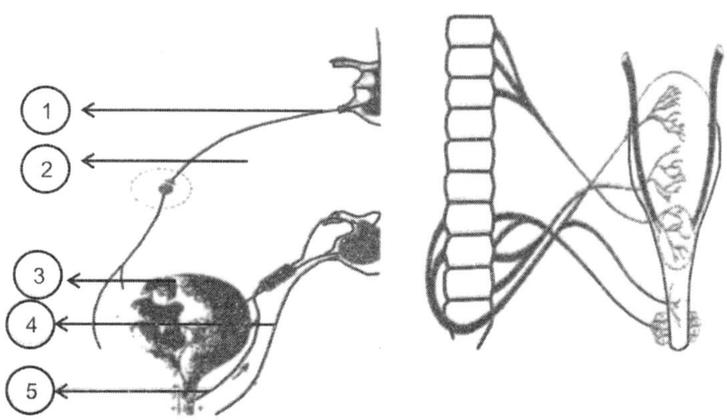

1. Identify 1, 2, 3, 4, 5.
2. Which nerve is called nerve of filling and nerve of emptying and why?

COMMENT/ANSWER

Innervation of Urinary Bladder

1. 1–Presynaptic sympathetic fibres from the lumbar segments, 2–Hypogastric ganglion, 3–Urinary bladder, 4–Parasympathetic afferent and efferent nerves from the lumbar segments, 5–Internal urethra.
2. Sympathetic fibres are called the nerve of filling parasympathetic fibres are called the nerve of emptying. Stimulation of the sympathetic fibres produces relaxation of the detrusor muscle and contraction of the internal urethral sphincter and parasympathetic stimulation causes the opposite effect.

28

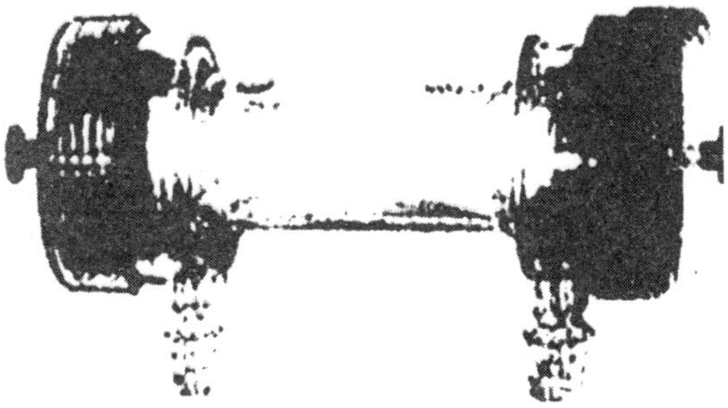

1. Identify the picture.
2. Which solute is significantly low in the dialysing fluid in comparison to the uremic plasma ?

COMMENT/ANSWER

Dialyser

1. Dialyser or artificial kidney, chronic renal failure.
2. Potassium.

29

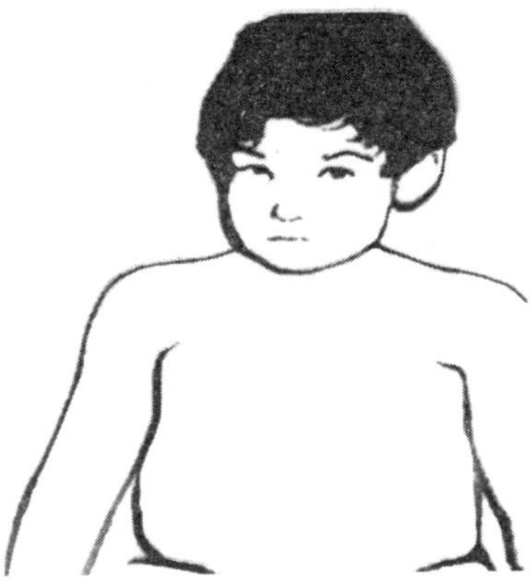

1. Identify the above condition.
2. Give any two characteristic features of the above condition.

COMMENT/ANSWER

1. Nephrotic syndrome.
2. Causes are:
   i. Hypoproteinemia.
   ii. Albuminuria.
   Hypocholesterolemia.

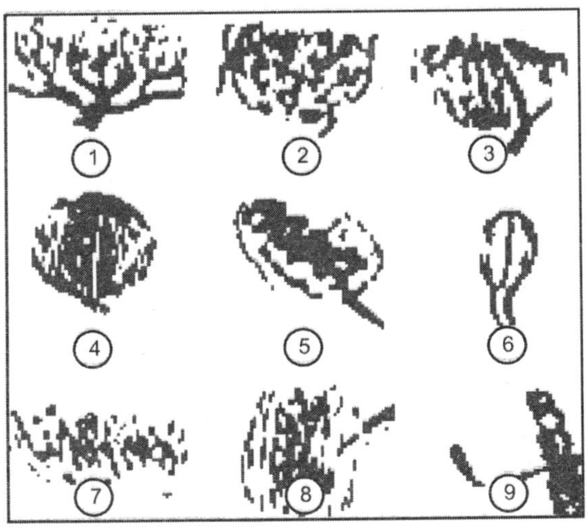

30

1. Identify 1 to 9.
2. Name the potential developed in these structures.
3. Enumerate at least 3 properties of these structures.

COMMENT/ANSWER

Receptors

1. 1–Free nerve endings, 2–Expanded tip receptor, 3–Tactile hair, 4–Pacinian corpuscle, 5–Meissner's corpuscle, 6–Krause corpuscle, 7–Ruffini's end–organ, 8–Golgi tendon apparatus, 9–Muscle spindle
2. Generator potential
3. 1–Specificity of response, 2–Adaptation, 3–Response increases to an increase in logarithm of intensity of stimulus. (Weber-Fechner's law)

31

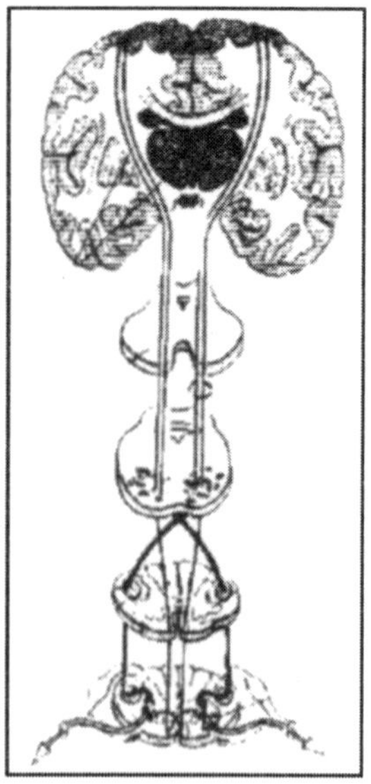

1. Identify this tract.
2. What is the function of this tract?
3. What is the commonest site? Where this tract gets damaged and what clinical features does it produce?

COMMENT/ANSWER

Pyramidal Tract

1. The pyramidal tract.
2. This is the tract which initiates voluntary motor impulses from the precentral gyrus.
3. The commonest site where this tract is damaged is at the internal capsule. Features of pyramidal tract disease include:
   a. Loss of voluntary motor function.
   b. Hypertonia.
   c. Absent superficial reflexes.
   d. Exaggerated deep tendon reflexes.
   e. Clonus.
   f. Babinski's sign positive.

32

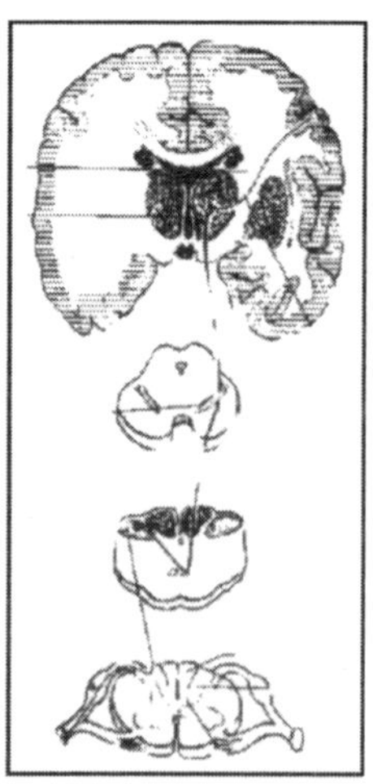

1. Identify this tract. What is the other name for this tract?
2. What are the sensations carried by this tract?

COMMENT/ANSWER

Dorsal Column

1. Dorsal column which are also known as the tracts of gracilis and cuneatus or tract of Goll and Burdach.
2. a. Conscious proprioception
   b. Joint and position sense
   c. Vibration sense
   d. Fine touch including tactile localization and tactile discrimination.
   e. Stereognosis.
   f. Pressure.

33

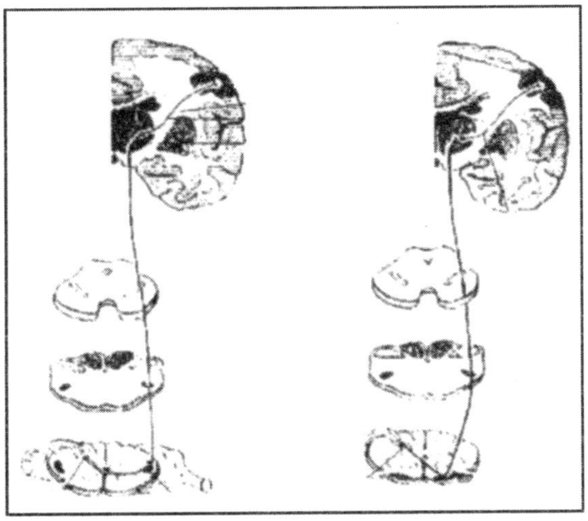

1. Identify the tracts.
2. What are the sensations carried by these tracts?

COMMENT/ANSWER

Lateral and Ventral Spinothalamic Tracts

1. Lateral and ventral spinothalamic tracts.
2. The lateral spinothalamic tract carries pain and temperature sensations while the ventral spinothalamic tract carries crude touch sensation.

34

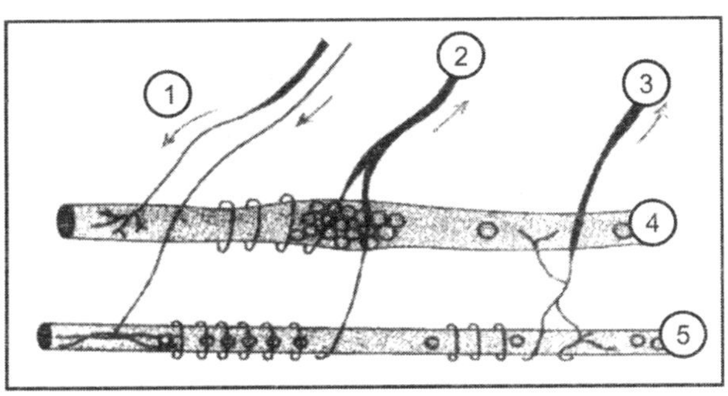

1. Identify 1, 2, 3, 4, 5.
2. What is the function of each structure?

COMMENT/ANSWER

Muscle Spindle

1. 1–Gamma efferent, 2–Group Ia primary afferent, 3–Group II secondary afferent, 4–Nuclear bag fibre, 5–Nuclear chain fiber
2. Muscle spindle is a proprioceptor which plays a very important role in myotatic (stretch) reflex and also responsible for sending information to the nervous system depicting the muscle length or rate of change of its length.

35

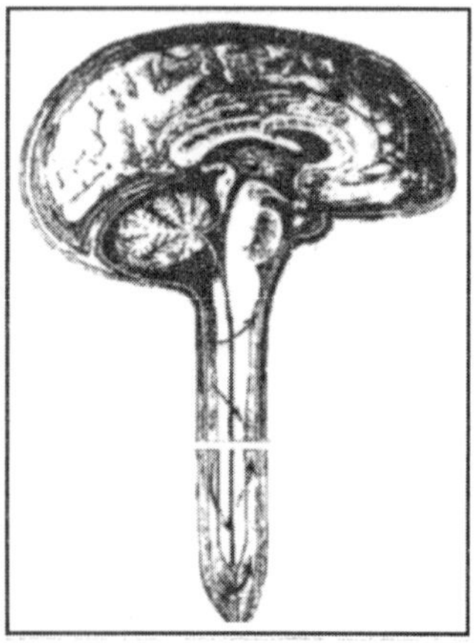

1. Identify the structure.
2. What is the normal CSF pressure? How is CSF analysis useful?

COMMENT/ANSWER

Circulation of CSF

1. The above structure represents the sagittal section of the brain, ventricles, spinal cord and meninges showing the circulation of CSF in the central nervous system.
2. The normal CSF pressure recorded by a lumbar puncture with the subject in the supine position is about 7–20 cm H_2O.
3. CSF analysis helps to:
   a. Diagnose and manage CNS infections, e.g. tuberculosis meningitis.
   b. Diagnose subarachnoid hemorrhage.
   c. Diagnose inflammatory disease of the CNS, e.g. multiple sclerosis.

36

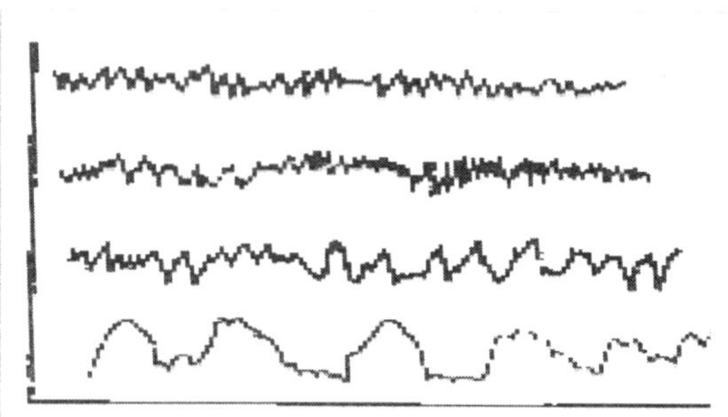

1. Identify the various waves and mention the cycles.
2. What are the uses of this curve?
3. What waves are seen during second stage is NREM and REM?

COMMENT/ANSWER

Electroencephalogram

1. This recording is called electroencephalogram.
   1. Alpha waves—frequency 8–13 cycles per sec.
   2. Beta waves—frequency 14–30 cycles per sec.
   3. Theta waves—frequency 4–7 cycles per sec.
   4. Delta waves—frequency 0.5–3–5 cycles per sec.
2. The uses of EEG are:
   1. To diagnose epilepsy, subdural hematoma and other brain disorders.
   2. In medicolegal cases.
   3. To guide in the prognosis of treatment of epilepsy.
   4. In neurophysiological studies.
3. The waves seen during the stage of REM–beta waves NREM—theta waves.

37

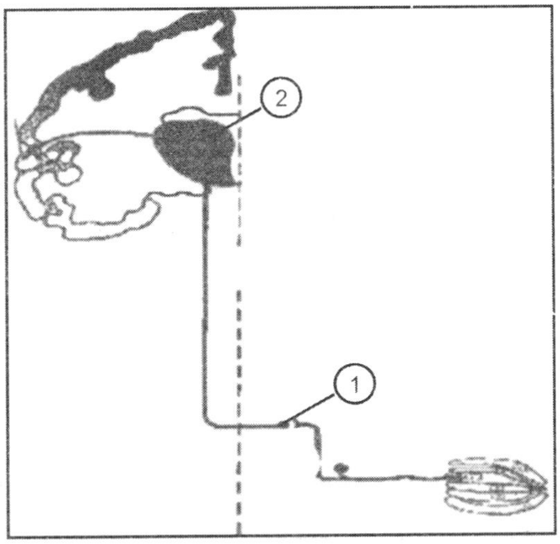

1. Name 1, 2.
2. What are the primary taste sensation?
3. Where do they take pathway in the brain?

COMMENT/ANSWER

Taste Pathway

1. 1–Nucleus of tractus solitarius
   2–Ventral posterolateral nucleus of thalamus.
2. The primary taste sensations are sweet, salt, sour and bitter.
3. This pathway terminates in the:
   1. Foot of postcentral gyrus.
   2. Anterior part of insula.

38

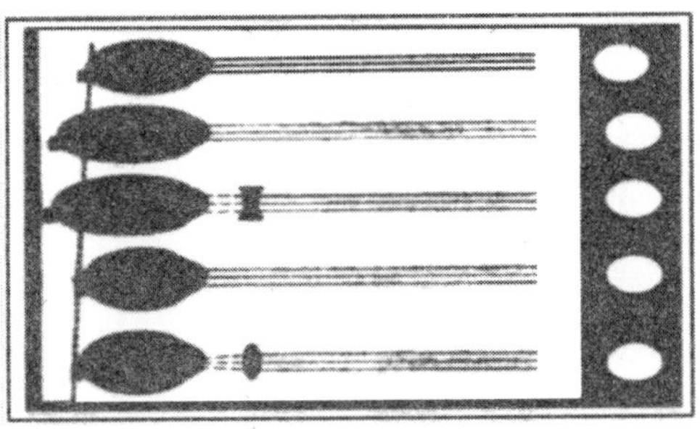

1. Which is the normal and abnormal eye?
2. What type of refractive error is seen in B and D and why?
3. What type of correction is made for the above errors and identify?

COMMENT/ANSWER

1. A–Normal eye, B and D–Abnormal eyes
2. B and D are abnormal eyes with myopia and hypermetropia, respectively. Cause of myopia—anteroposterior diameter is long. Hypermetropia anteroposterior diameter is short.
3. Myopia—divertgent lens—biconcave lens. Hypermetropia—convergent lens—biconvex lens.

39

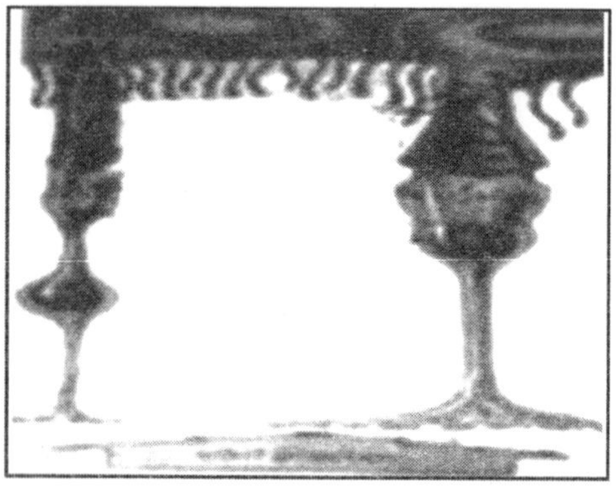

1. Identify 1 and 2.
2. What is the function of 1 and 2?
3. When does function of structure 1 better?
4. When does function of structure 2 better?

COMMENT/ANSWER

Rod and Cone

1. 1–Rod, 2–Cone.
2. The function of rods and cones is that they act as visual receptors for both dimlight and dark vision.
3. Rods function better during dimlight or night vision.
4. Cones function better during bright light for acuity and also for color vision.

40

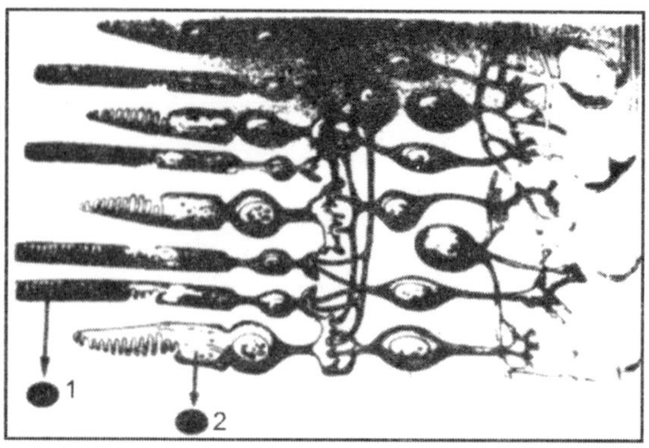

1. Identify 1 and 2.
2. What potential is developed at this structure ?
3. What is the function of 1 and 2? Mention three differences between them.

COMMENT/ANSWER

Rods and Cones

1. Rods and cones.
2. Hyperpolarisation potential.
3. Rods carry impulses mediating black and white vision while cones carry impulses mediating color and bright vision.
   - Rods mediate scotopic vision while cones mediate photopic vision.
   - There are 120 million rods and 6 million cones.
   - Rods are more sensitive than cones to stimulation by light.

41

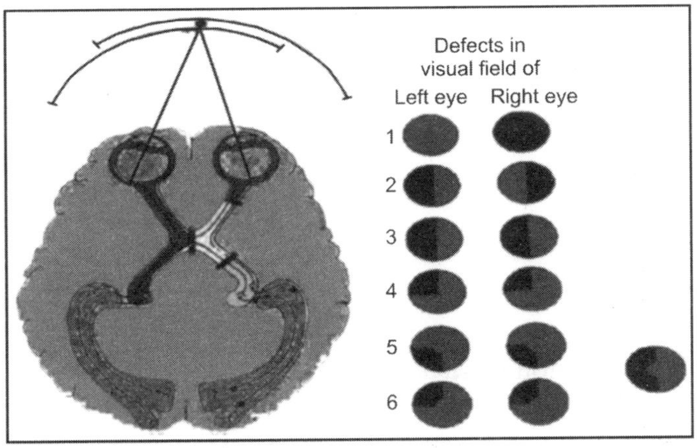

1. Trace this pathway from its origin to its termination
2. Name the visual areas of cerebral cortex
3. What happens when there is lesion at the level of medial fibres crossing at optic chiasma?

COMMENT/ANSWER

Visual Pathway

1. Optic nerve–optic chiasma–optic tract–lateral geniculate body–geniculocalcarine radiations–visual cortex.
2. Broadman's visual area–area 17. Visual association area–areas 18, 19.
3. Bitemporal heteronymous hemianopia.

42

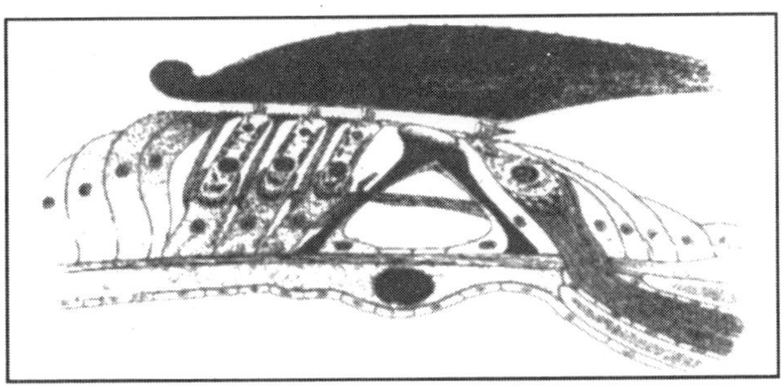

1. Identify the structure.
2. What type of potential is developed at this area?
3. Name the theories of hearing.

COMMENT/ANSWER

Organ of Corti

1. Cross-section of cochlea shows the organ of corti.
2. Endocochlear potential.
   Cochlear microphonic potential.
   Action potential of auditory nerve.
3. Rutherford telephone theory.
   Wever-Place theory.
   Helmholtz-Resonance-Volley theory.
   Von Bekesy's travelling wave theory.

43

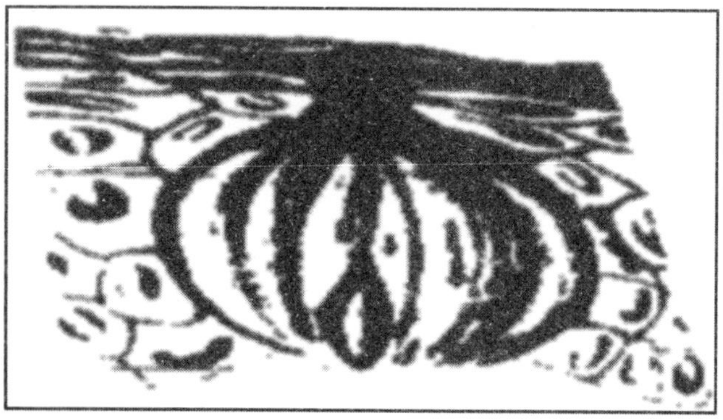

1. Identify the parts 1, 2 and 3.
2. Name the four primary taste sensations.
3. What is aguesia? Mention two causes for this condition.

COMMENT/ANSWER

Taste Bud

1. 1–Taste bud showing the taste pore, 2–Gustatory cell, 3–Supporting cells.
2. Sweet, sour, bitter and salt.
3. Loss of taste is known as aguesia. Common cold and fever for more than 3 days are the commonest cause of aguesia.

44

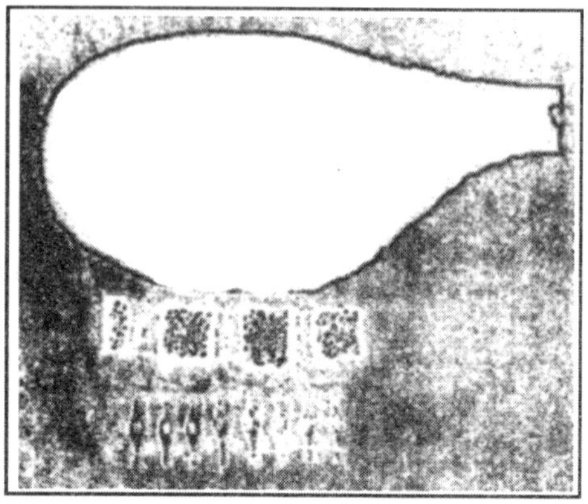

1. Identify the pathway.
2. What is the peculiar feature of this sensation?
3. What does this sensation termination in the cortex?
4. What is anosmia? Name two conditions producing anosmia.

COMMENT/ANSWER

1. Olfactory receptor with innervation.
2. Peculiar features:
   i. Most vestigial of all senses.
   ii. Does not pass through thalamus. But an alternate pathway has been recently discovered that is claimed to pass via thalamus.
3. Uncus of parahippocampal gyrus.
4. Anosmia: Loss of sensation of smell. Two causes: 1. Coryza (common cold), 2. Viral rhinitis (influenza), allergic rhinitis

45

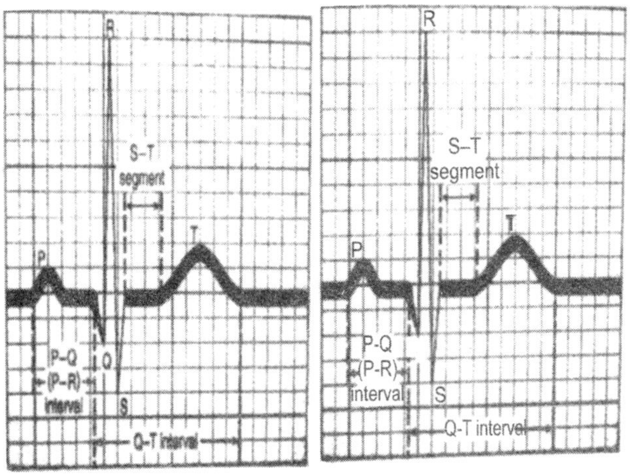

1. What is PR interval?
2. What is the cause for PR interval?
3. How will you calculate the heart rate ?

COMMENT/ANSWER

ECG

1. This is an electrocardiogram. PR interval is the interval between the beginning of P wave and beginning of R wave.
2. *Cause:* The time taken for conduction of impulse from SA node to AV node producing atrial depolarization and AV nodal delay.
3. Heart rate= 1500/number of small squares between two subsequent R waves.(Or) Heart rate=300/ number of large squares between two subsequent R waves.

46

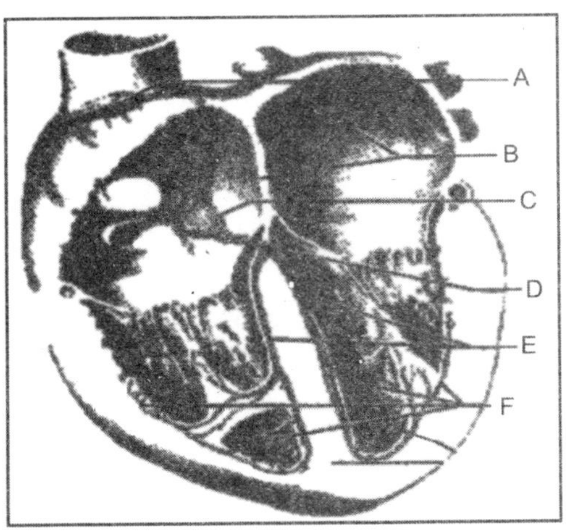

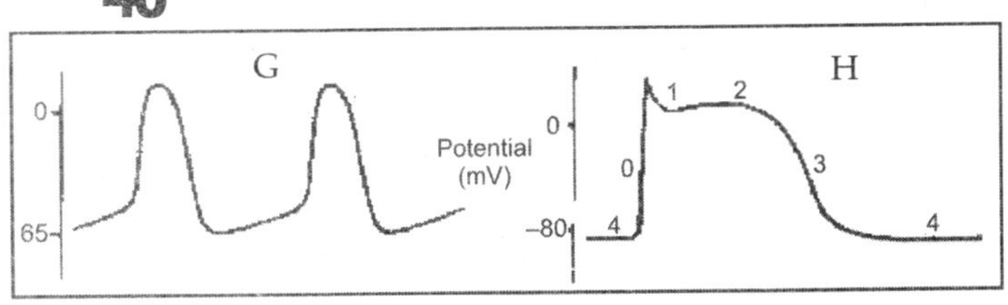

1. Identify this structure and name the A, B, C, D, E and F parts.
2. Name the G and H curves.
3. What is the Ionic basis of 1, 2, 3 of G curve and 0, 1, 2, 3 and 4 of H curve?

COMMENT/ANSWER

Conduction System with Action Potential

1. A. SA node', B. AV node, C. Bundle of His, D. Right and left bundle branches, E. Purkinje fibres, F. Ventricular wall
2. G. Membrane potential of pacemaker tissue.
   H. Membrane potential of ventricular muscle.
3. G–Curve:
   1. Ca^+ entry Na^+ entry K^+ efflux.
   2. Ca^+ entry.
   3. K^+ efflux.

   H – Curve:

   0 – Na^+ influx

   1. K^+ efflux and Cl influx
   2. Ca^+ influx through show channels.
   3. Rapid K^+ efflux.
   4. Restoration of RMP due to K^+ efflux.

47

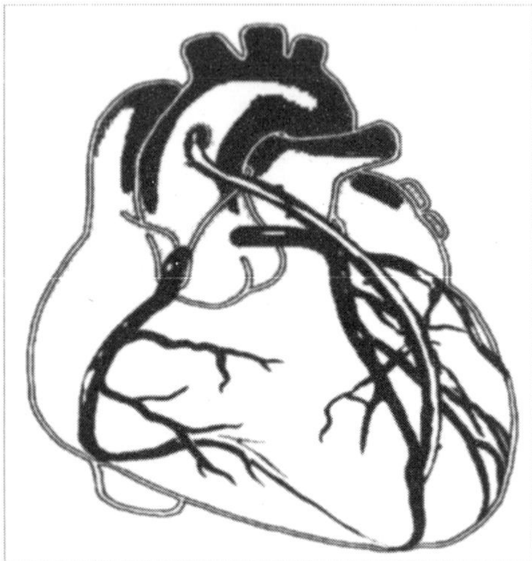

1. Identify the picture
2. What are the peculiar features of coronary circulation?

COMMENT/ANSWER

Coronary Circulation

1. Coronary circulation.
2. i. They are end arteries.
   ii. It is the only organ in which maximum flow is received during diastole (phasic flow).
   iii. Heart is the only organ of the body that generates its own perfusion pressure (by autoregulation).
   iv. They have a high oxygen extraction ratio.

48

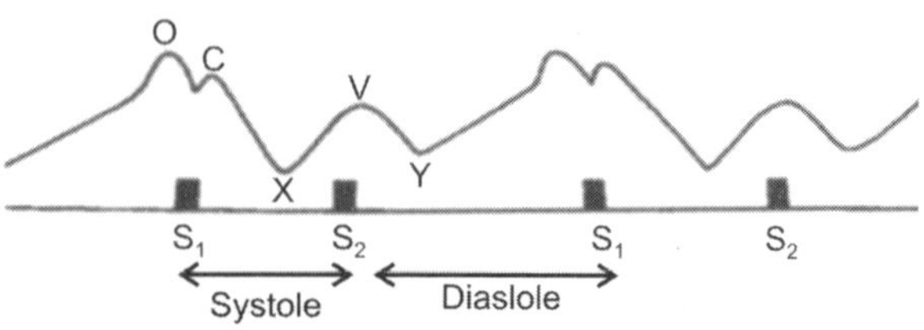

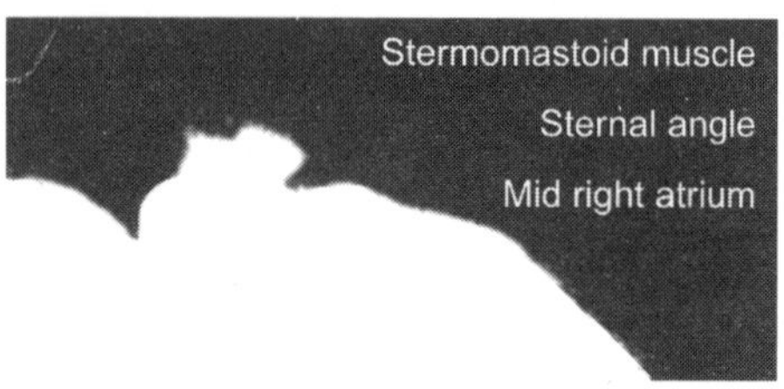

1. Identify the curve.
2. Name the bar below the curve and its cause.
3. Why right side of the neck is always examined for jugular venous pulse?
4. Give the cause for each wave in the above curve.

COMMENT/ANSWER

Jugular Venous Pulse

1. The curve is a jugular venous pulse tracing.
2. The bar below indicates the heart sounds. The cause of S1—closure of atrioventricular valves. S2—closure of semilunar valves.
3. Jugular venous is examined on the right side because:
   1. It is in direct line with the right atrium.
   2. There are no valves in the jugular vein and hence the activity of the right atrium is best seen on the right side. Jugular vein is not hidden by many facial planes and so not obliterated.
4. a wave denotes atrial systole.
   c wave denotes rise in atrial pressure during isometric contraction period.
   x wave denotes atrial diastole and start of ventricular systole.
   v wave denotes increases in pressure due to filling of atria.
   y wave denotes fall in pressure due to the opening of atrioventricular valves.

49

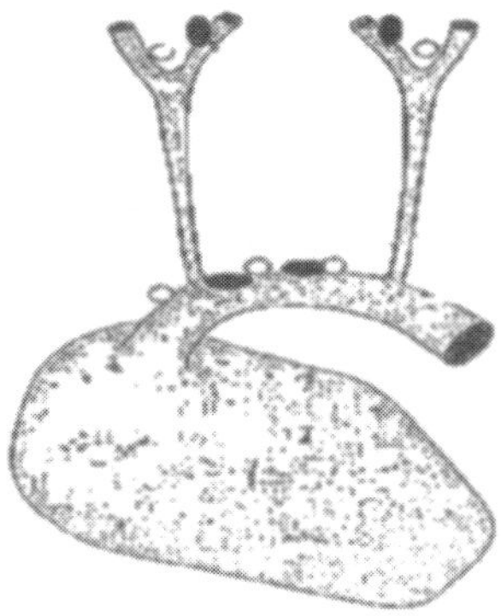

1. Identify 1 and 2 ?
2. Where are they situated?
3. What is the function of 1 and 2? What is Cushing's reflex ?

COMMENT/ANSWER

Baroreceptors

1. 1–Carotid body, 2–Aortic body
2. Carotid body is situated at the bifurcation of the common carotid artery. Aortic body is at the external arch of aorta.
3. They function as chemoreceptors and respond to hypoxia, hypercapnea, and acidosis. Cushing's reflex: When BP falls below 40 mm Hg due to ischemia of the brain, there is direct stimulation of VMC leading to rise in BP with bradycardia. It is the last ditch effort.

50

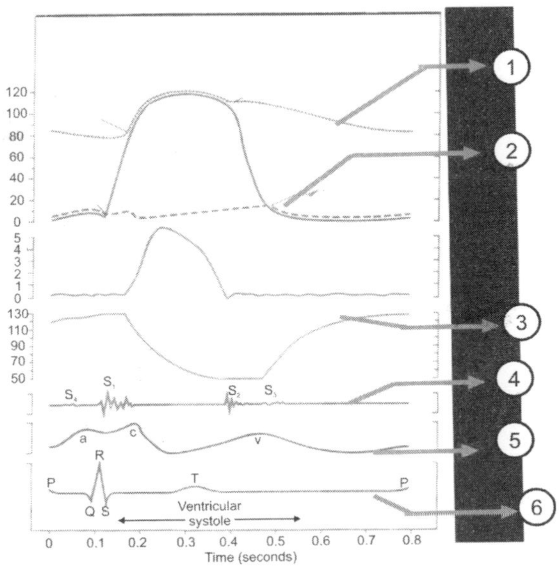

1. Identify the various curves 1–6 and name them.
2. Correlate the ECG recording with heart sounds.
3. What is phonocardiogram and echocardiogram?

COMMENT/ANSWER

Cardiac Cycle

1. Cardiac cycle event
   1. Aortic pressure curve.
   2. Ventricular pressure curve.
   3. Ventricular volume curve.
   4. Heart sounds (phonocardiogram).
   5. Jugular venous pressure curve.
   6. Electrocardiogram.
2. 1st heart sound—closure of atrioventricular valves. 2nd heart sound—closure of semilunar valves.
3. Phonocardiogram—recording of heart sounds. Echocardiogram—an ultrasonic record obtained by echocardiography. Used in the diagnosis of cardiovascular lesions and recording of the size, motion and composition of various cardiac structures.

51

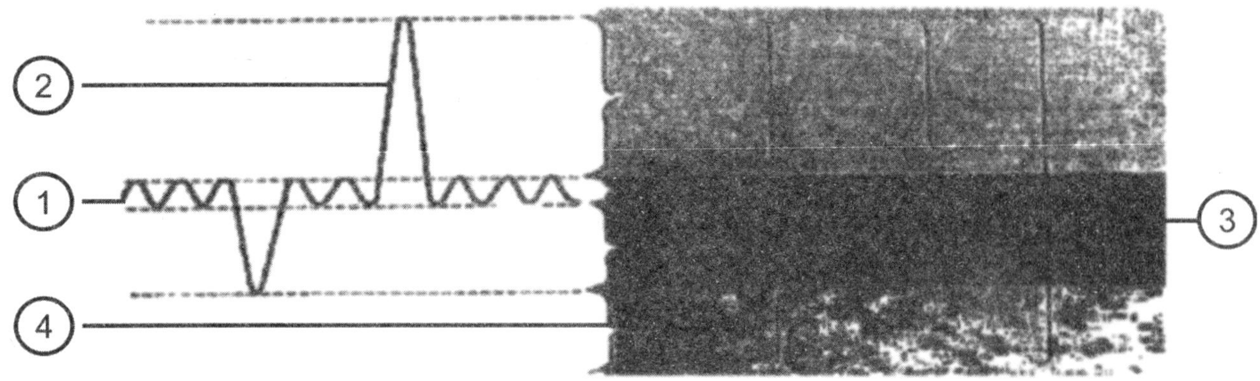

1. Identify 1, 2, 3, 4. Give definition of each.
2. What is the function of FRC and explain.
3. Mention the name of two methods to measure FRC.

COMMENT/ANSWER

1. 1–*Tidal volume:* The volume of air breathed in and out of the lung in a single normal respiration(500 ml).

   2–*Inspiratory capacity:* It is the maximum volume of air that can be inspired starting from end expiratory position. IC = TV + IRV = 500 + 3300 = 3800 ml.

   3–*Vital capacity:* It is the maximum amount of air that can be expelled out forcefully after a deep inspiration.
   VC = IRV + TV + ERV = 3300 + 500 + 1000 = 4800 ml.

   4–*Functional residual capacity:* It is the volume of air remaining in the lungs after normal expiration.
   FRC = ERV + RV = 1000 + 1200 = 2200 ml

2. Function of FRC:
   1. Helps in continuous exchange of gases between lungs and blood between two breath.
   2. Helps to prevent marked rise or fall in concentration of O_2 and CO_2 levels between inspiration and expiration.
3. The methods to find FRC are:
   1. Helium dilution technique.
   2. Nitrogen washout method.

52

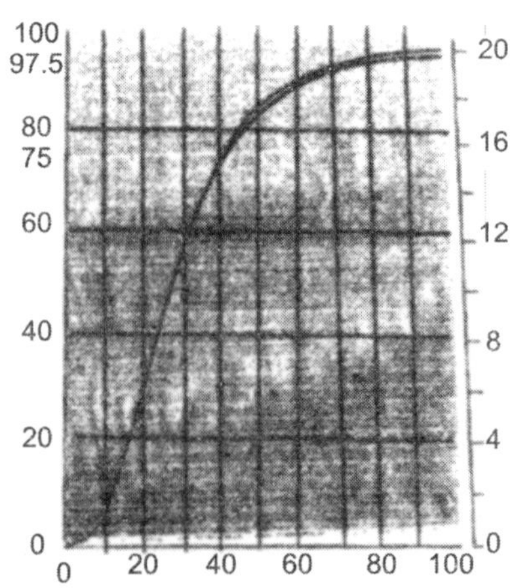

1. Identify the curve.
2. What is the effect of 2, 3 DPG on this curve?

COMMENT/ANSWER

1. This curve is an oxygen dissociation curve.
2. The effect of 2, 3 DPG is to shift the oxygen dissociation curve towards the right.

53

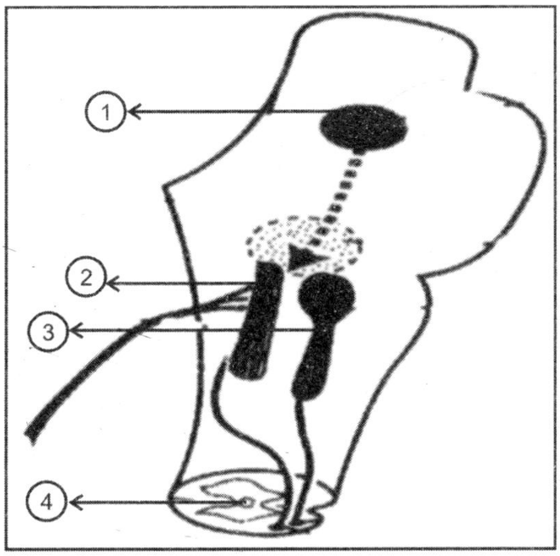

1. Identify 1, 2, 3, 4 and 5.
2. Which receptor in the lungs stimulate the respiratory centre.
3. What is inspiratory ramp signal? Where is it generated?

COMMENT/ANSWER

Regulation of Respiration

1. 1–Pneumotaxic centre in upper pons.
   2–Dorsal group of neurons.
   3–Ventral group of neurons.
   4–Vagus and glossopharyngeal nerves.
   5–Respiratory motor pathways
2. J receptor, irritant receptor, stretch receptor, chemoreceptor, joint receptor (proprioceptor).
3. Ramp signal is the inspiratory signal that increases in a ramp-like fashion for 2 sec and then ceases with immediate expiration for 3 sec. It is initiated in the dorsal group of neurons.

54

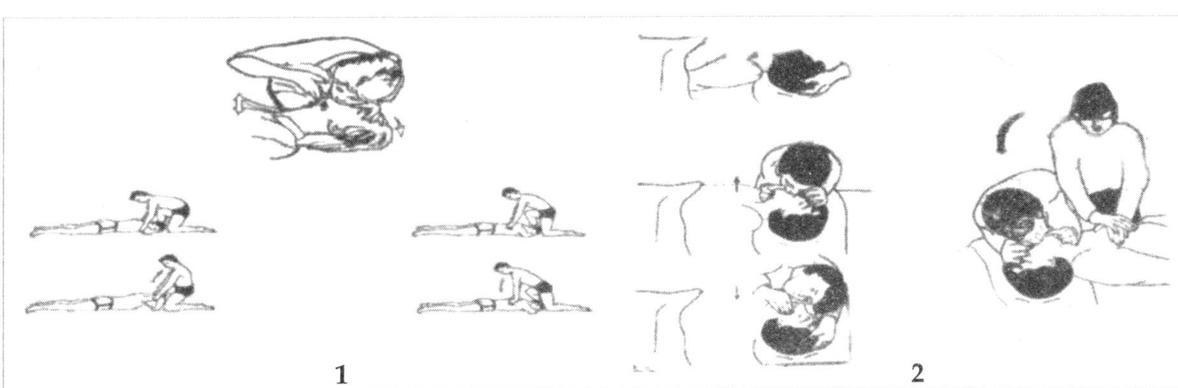

1. Identify 1 and 2.
2. What are the precautions taken during an artificial respiration?
3. Which is the best method? Why?

COMMENT/ANSWER

Artificial Respiration

1. These procedures are done for manual methods in artificial respiration.
   1–Mouth to mouth breathing
   2–Holger-Neilson method
2. To ensure that the airway is clear.
   Tongue should be drawn out.
   Tight cloths should be loosened.
   Patient should not be vomiting
3. This is the best method because the carbon dioxide in the expired air from the resuscitator can directly stimulate the respiratory centres and facilitate the onset of rhythmic respiration .

55

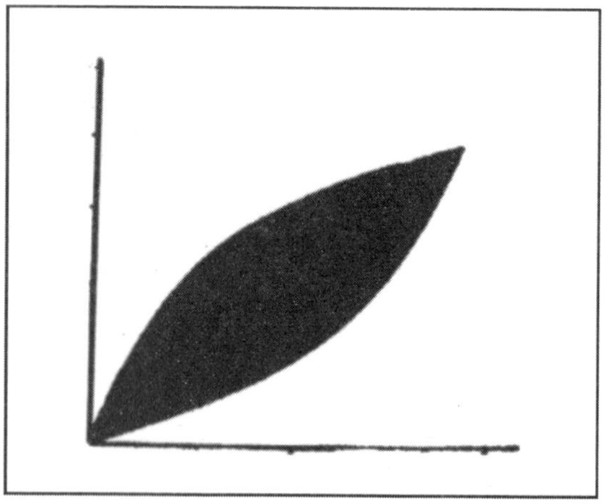

1. Identify the curve.
2. What is its normal value for the lung, thoracic cage and lungs together?
3. Name one condition where this value increases.

COMMENT/ANSWER

1. This is known as the compliance curve.
2. Lung compliance = 0.22 L/cm H_2O
   Lung and thoracic compliance = 0.13 L/cm H_2O
3. Compliance increases in emphysema and decreases in pulmonary fibrosis.

56

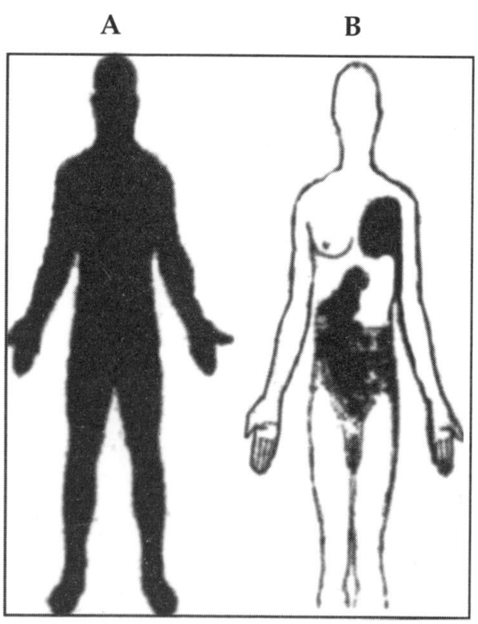

1. Identify these two pictures and what is the applied feature?
2. Give four classical examples.
3. What are the theories behined this phenomenon?

COMMENT/ANSWER

Referred Pain

1. Dermatome—the applied aspect of this picture is referred pain.
2. Left sholder pain—cardiac anginal pain
   Umblical pain—appendix and ovary pathology.
   Scrotal pain—ureteric colic.
   Right shoulder pain—right diaphragm irritation, gallbladder pathology.
3. Convergence and facilitation theory.

CALCULATION 1

The patient has the following haemogram values:

Hb = 14 gm%
RBC = 4 million/mm^3
PCV = 35%

1. Calculate MCV and MCH
2. Write the normal range of MCV and MCH.

Answer

$$MCV = \frac{PCV}{RC} \times 100$$
$$= \frac{35}{4} \times 10$$
$$= 87.5 \text{ (or) } 88\ \mu^3$$
$$MCH = \frac{Hb}{RBC} \times 10$$
$$= \frac{14}{4} \times 10$$
$$= 35Pg.$$

1. MCV is the average volume of a red blood cell. MCH is the amount of haemoglobin that is present in red blood cell.
2. Normal value MCV = 80 – 96 cubic microns.
   MCH = 27 – 30 Pg.

CALCULATION 2

The patient has the following haemogram values:

Hb = 7 gm%
RBC = 2 million/mm^3
PCV = 20%

1. Calculate MCHC and CI
2. Define MCHC. What is the normal range?

Answer

$$MCHC = \frac{Hb}{PCV} \times 100$$
$$= \frac{7}{20} \times 100$$
$$= 35\%$$
$$CI = \frac{Hb}{RBC} \times 100$$
$$= \frac{\frac{7}{15} \times 100}{\frac{2}{5} \times 100} = 1.16$$

1. *MCHC:* It is the average concentration of haemoglobin in 100 ml of blood.
   Normal range: MCHC = 32 to 36%
   Color index = 0.9 – 1.1

CALCULATION 3

Calculate the filtration fraction from the following data:

Glomerular filtration rate = 125 ml/min.
Renal plasma flow = 650 ml/min.

1. Name the various pressures contributing to filtration process?
2. What are their normal values?

Answer

Filtration fraction = GFR/renal plasma flow
= 125/650
= 0.19

1. Hydrostatic pressure of the glomerular capillaries, osmotic pressure in the glomerular capillaries, hydrostatic pressures of the Bowman's capsule are the various pressures involved in glomerular filtration.
2. Hydrostatic pressure of the glomerular capillaries = 60 mmHg
   Hydrostatic pressure of the Bowman's capsule = 18 mmHg
   Osmotic pressure of the fluid in the glomerular capillaries = 32 mmHg

CALCULATION 4

Calculate the inulin clearance:

Concentration of inulin in plasma = 1 mg/ml
Concentration of inulin in urine = 127 mg/ml
Volume of urine excreted per minute = 1 ml

1. What does this clearance indicate?
2. What other clearances indicate GFR?

Answer

$$\text{Inulin clearance} = UV/P$$
$$= \frac{127}{1} \times 1$$
$$= 127 \text{ ml/min.}$$

1. This clearance indicates the normal GFR. Creatinine clearance and 51Cr EDTA–radio isotopes are the other clearances indicating GFR.

CALCULATION 5

Calculate the renal plasma flow with the following data:

Venous plasma level of PAH is = 0.1 mg
Concentration of PAH in Urine = 66 mg
The volume of urine output = 1 ml/min.

1. What is the normal renal plasma flow?
2. What other substance that can be used to measure this?

Answer

$$\text{Renal plasma flow} = \frac{UV}{P}$$

$$= \frac{\text{Concentration of PAH in urine} \times \text{Volume of urine output}}{\text{Venous plasma level of PAH}}$$

$$= \frac{66}{0.1} \times 1 = 660 \text{ mg/min.}$$

1. Normal renal plasma flow is 625 ml/min.
2. The other substance used to measure renal plasma flow is diodrast.

CALCULATION 6

Calculate the renal plasma flow with the following data:

Venous plasma level of PAH is = 0.02 mg/ml
Urine PAH level is = 12 mg/ml
Urine flow is = 1 ml/min.

1. What is the normal renal plasma flow?
2. What other substance can be used to measure this?
3. Mention two peculiar features of renal circulation?

Answer

Renal plasma flow = UV/P
= 12 × 1/0.02
= 600 ml/min.

1. 650 ml.
2. Diodrast is the other substance used measure renal plasma flow.
3. a. Renal arteries arise directly from abdominal aorta and hence it has a higher renal hydrostatic pressure of 60 mmHg.
   b. Kidneys receives maximum blood flow, about 1200 ml of blood/min.
   c. Renal circulation has a portal system that is a double network of capillaries.
      a. Afferent arteriole → Glomerular capillaries
      b. Efferent arteriole → Peritubular capillaries
   d. Autoregulation of blood flow is well established in kidneys in the range (80–180 mmHg).

CALCULATION 7

Calculate the GFR from the following data:

Concentration of plasma inulin = 0.3 mg/ml
Concentration of urine inulin = 12.3 mg/ml
Urine flow = 3 ml/min

If diodrast clearance is 738 ml/min, calculate the filtration fraction.

1. Define filtration fraction and filtration coefficient?
2. Mention their normal values?

Answer

GFR = UV/P
= 12.3 × 3/0.3
= 123 ml/min

Filtration fraction = GFR/RPF = 123/738 = 0.16

1. **Filtration fraction** is the fraction of plasma that is filtered. It is the ratio of glomerular filtration rate to renal plasma flow. **Filtration coefficient** is the ratio of glomerular filtration rate to effective filtration pressure.
2. **Normal value**
   Filtration fraction = 0.19
   Filtration coefficient = 12.5 ml/min/mm Hg

CALCULATION 8

Calculate the total body water from the following data:

Amount of D_2O injected = 100 ml
Amount of D_2O excreted in one hour = 4 ml
Plasma concentration of D_2O at the end of one hour = 0.002 ml/min

1. How is total body water divided in the body?

Answer

Total body water = Amount of (substance injected – substance excreted) plasma concentration of the substance

$$= \frac{100 - 4}{0.002}$$

= 48,000 ml (or) 48 lit.

Total body water is divided into extracellular fluid and intracellular fluid. Again ECF is divided into interstitial fluid and plasma.

CALCULATION 9

Calculate the total body water from the following data:
Amount of D_2O injected = 80 ml.
Amount of D_2O excreted in one hour = 3 ml.
Plasma concentration of D_2O at the end of one hour = 0.002 ml/min.

1. How is total body water measured?
2. Give examples of transcellular fluid?

Answer

Total body water = Amount of (substance injected – substance excreted) plasma concentration of the substance

$$= \frac{80-3}{0.002} = 38500 \text{ ml (or) } 38.5 \text{ lit.}$$

1. Indicator dilution method is used to measure total body water. Substances used are T_3O and antipyrine.
2. Some examples of transcellular fluid are pericardial fluid, peritoneal fluid, CSF, synovial fluid, aqueous humour, etc.

CALCULATION 10

Calculate the extracellular fluid volume from the following data:
Amount of thiocyanate injected = 400 mg
Amount of thiocyanate excreted in 1 hour = 30 mg
Plasma thiocyanate concentration at the end of one hour = 3.8 mg%

1. Name the physiological and pathological conditions in which extracellular fluid volume increases and decreases?

Answer

$$\text{EFC} = \frac{400-30}{3.8} \times 100 = 9737 \text{ ml} = 10 \text{ lit}$$

Physiological
Increased ECF
1. Pregnancy

Pathological
Increased ECF
1. Over hydration due to excess ADH
2. Water intoxication

Physiological
Decreased ECF
1. Excess sweating

Pathological
Decreased ECF
1. Diarrhoea
2. Vomiting
3. Over use of diuretics
4. Addison's diseases
5. Decreased ADH.

CALCULATION 11

Calculate the interstitial fluid volume from the following data:
Amount of inulin injected = 120 mg
Amount of inulin excreted in one hour = 5 mg
Plasma inulin concentration at the end of one hour = 0.01 mg/ml
Plasma volume = 3500 ml

1. How is the ECF different from intracellular fluid?

Answer

$$\text{ECF} = \frac{\text{Amount of injected subs tan ce} - \text{Amount of substance excreted}}{\text{Plasma concentration}}$$

$$= \frac{120-5}{0.01}$$

$$= \frac{115}{0.01}$$

$$= 11500 \text{ ml}$$

Interstitial fluid = ECF – Plasma volume
= 11500 – 3500
= 8000 ml

The extracellular fluid is different from intracellular fluid based on the ionic concentration in ECF. In ECF, sodium is the chief cation. Chloride and bicarbonate are the chief anions whereas in ICF, potassium is the predominant cation. Proteins and organic phosphates are predominant anions.

CALCULATION 12

Calculate the maximum urea clearance from the following data:
Blood urea concentration = 0.3 mg/ml
Urine urea concentration = 9 mg/ml
Urine flow = 2.4 ml/min

1. What is the difference between maximum and standard urea clearance? What are their normal values?

Answer

Maximum urea clearance = UV/P

$$= \frac{2.4 \times 9}{0.3}$$

1. **Maximum urea clearance:** Is determined when urine flow is more than 2 ml/min.

   Formula = $\frac{UV}{P}$

Standard urea clearance: Is determined when urine flow is less than 2 ml/min.

$$\text{Formula} = U \times \frac{\sqrt{V}}{P}$$

2. Maximum urea clearance = 72 ml/min.
   Standard urea clearance = 55 ml/min.

CALCULATION 13

A married woman with regular menstrual periods missed her periods from 3rd October 2003. Calculate her expected date of delivery?

1. What is the normal duration of pregnancy?
2. When does ovulation occur?
3. Define menorrhagia, amenorrhoea, dysmenorrhoea, oligomenorrhoea, premenstrual tension?

Answer

The expected date of delivery is 10.07.2004 (+7 days and – 3 months)

1. 280 days
2. Ovulation occur on 14th day of menstrual cycle
3. *Menorrhagia:* Is excess menstrual bleeding

   Amenorrhoea: Is absence of menstrual bleeding

   Dysmenorrhoea: Is painful menstruation

   Oligomenorrhoea: Is reduced menstrual bleeding

   Premenstrual tension: Is pain in lower abdomen before menstruation.

CALCULATION 14

Calculate the respiratory quotient from the data given below:

Volume of expired air in 6 min = 30 L
Percentage of carbon dioxide in expired air = 4.2%
Oxygen consumption in 6 min = 1470 ml

1. What is the normal oxygen consumption/min by our body?
2. Under what situation does oxygen consumption increase?

Answer

Volume of expired air in 6 min = 30 L/6
Volume of expired air in 1 min = 5 L
% of carbon dioxide in expired air = 4.2%
Therefore of carbon dioxide in min contain

$$= 500 \times \frac{4.2}{100} = 210 \text{ ml of } CO_2$$

O_2 consumed in 6 min = 1470 ml

Therefore O_2 consumed in 1 min $= \frac{1470}{6}$

$$\text{Respiratory quotient} = \frac{CO_2 \text{ output/min}}{O_2 \text{ consumed/min}}$$

$$= \frac{210}{245} = 0.85$$

1. 250 ml/min
2. 1–Exercise, 2–Fever, 3–Hyperthroidism.

CALCULATION 15

Calculate the alveolar ventilation using the following data:

Tidal volume - 500 ml
Dead space - 150 ml
Respiratory rate - 12/min

1. What is V/Q ratio? What is its normal value?
2. What are the uses of dead space?

Answer

Alveolar ventilation = (Tidal volume – Dead space) × Respiratory rate
= (500 – 150) × 12
= 4200 ml/min

1. V/Q ratio is the ratio of alveolar ventilation to the perfusion of blood to the alveolus. Normal value = 0.8
2. Functions of dead space.
   i. Responsible for filtration of dust particles.
   ii. Humidification of air.
   iii. Brings the expired air to normal body temperature.

CALCULATION 16

Calculate the breathing reserve and the dyspneic index:

Maximum voluntary ventilation = 80 L/min
Pulmonary ventilation = 7 L/min

1. Below what values of dyspneic index does the subject develop dyspnoea?
2. Name the commonest cause of dyspnoea in the respiratory system and cardiovascular system.

Answer

$$\text{Breathing reserve} = \frac{(MVV - PC)}{(MVV)} \times 100$$

$$= \frac{80 - 7}{80} \times 100$$

$$= \frac{7300}{80}$$

$$= 91\%$$

1. 65%
2. Commonest cause of dyspnoea in respiratory—bronchial asthma, chronic bronchitis, emphysema. Cardiovascular condition—congestive cardiac failure.

CALCULATION 17

Calculate the dead space with following values.

Area with N_2 - 70 sq.cm.
Area without N_2 - 30 sq.cm
The volume of air - 500 ml

1. What is dyspnoea, apnoea, eupnoea, tachypnoea, bradypnea, paroxysmal nocturnal dyspnoea?

Answer

$$\text{Dead space} = \frac{\text{Area without } N_2 \times \text{Volume of air}}{\text{Area with } N_2 + \text{Area without } N_2}$$

$$= \frac{30 \times 500}{70 + 30}$$

$$= 150 \text{ ml}$$

1. *Dyspnoea:* Difficulty in breathing where the solicit is conscious of shortness of breath.
   Apnoea: Temporary cessation of breathing
   Eupnoea: Normal pattern of respiration
   Tachypnoea: Increase in the rate of breathing
   Bradypnoea: Decrease in the rate of breathing
   Paroxysmal noctural dyspnoea: Attacks of severe dyspnoea occurring at nights.

CALCULATION 18

Calculate the functional residual capacity from the following data:

Volume of air collected	-	40 lit.
Concentration of N_2 in collected air	-	5 %
Normal concentration of N_2 in air	-	80%

1. What is the normal value of residual volume and functional residual capacity?
2. What is the function of functional residual capacity? How is it measured?

Answer

$$\text{Functional residual capacity} = V \times C1/C2 = \frac{40000 \times 5/100}{80/100} = 2500 \text{ ml}$$

1. RV = 1200 ml
   FRC = 2500 ml
   i. Helps in continues exchange of gases between lungs and blood between two breaths.
   ii. Helps to prevent marked rise or fall in concentration of oxygen and carbon dioxide level between inspiration and expiration.
2. FRC is measured by:
   1. Helium dilution method
   2. Nitrogen washout method.

CALCULATION 19

In a pulmonary function test, the following data are obtained:

Vital capacity	=	4.5 lit
Expiratory reserve volume	=	1.3 lit
N_2 alveolar air	=	80%
Total volume of expired air N_2	=	28 lit
After complete N_2 washout		
Concentration of N_2 in collected air	=	4%

Calculate functional residual capacity, residual volume and total lung capacity.

1. What are the normal values of functional residual capacity, residual volume and total lung capacity?
2. How is functional residual capacity measured?

$$FRC = \frac{N_2 \text{ in collected air} \times \text{Total volume of expired air}}{N_2 \text{ in alveolar air}}$$

$$= \frac{4/100 \times 28000}{80/100} = 1400 \text{ ml}$$

Residual volume = FRC – ERV = 1400 – 1300 = 100 ml

Total lung capacity = VC + RV = 4500 + 100 = 4600 ml

1. FRC = 2500 ml, RV = 1200 ml, TLC = 6000 ml
2. FRC is measured by:
   1. Helium dilution method.
   2. Nitrogen washout method.

CALCULATION 20

Calculate the percentage of cardiac output going to the heart from the following data:

Heart rate	-	70/min
Stroke volume	-	72 ml
Blood flow to heart	-	195 ml/100 gm
Weight of heart	-	150 gm

1. What is the peculiar feature of blood flow to this organ?
2. What is the normal blood flow to this organ in one minute?

Answer

Cardiac output	= 70 × 72 = 5040 ml/min
Blood flow to heart	= 150 × 195/100 = 285 ml/min
% of cardiac output	= 285 × 100/5040 = 5.6%

1. i. Coronary arteries are end arteries.
   ii. Coronary circulation has high oxygen extraction ratio.
   iii. It has phasic blood flow.
2. 200 to 250 ml/min.

CALCULATION 21

Calculate the percentage of cardiac output going to the brain from the following data:

Heart rate	-	75/min
Stroke volume	-	62 ml
Blood flow to brain	-	100 ml/100 gm
Weight of brain	-	800 gm

1. What is the peculiar feature of blood flow to this organ?
2. What is the normal blood flow to this organ in one minute?

Answer

Cardiac output	= 75 × 62 = 4650 ml/min
Blood flow to brain	= 800 × 100/100
	= 800 ml/min
% of cardiac output	= 800 × 100/4650
	= 17%

1. The peculiar features of this blood flow to the brain are:
   i. Autoregulation is maintained between 65–140 mmHg.
   ii. The cerebral vascular resistance offered by increase in the intracranial pressure, CSF pressure and viscosity is high, the cerebral circulation is reduced.
   iii. Cushing reflex

   Increase in intracranial pressure reduces the blood flow for a short period. This blood flow is being re-established due to the activation of the vasomotor center, thereby increasing the blood pressure.
2. The normal blood flow is 200–250 ml/100 gm of substance.

CALCULATION 22

Calculate the percentage of cardiac output going to the skin from the following data:

Heart rate	-	72/min
Stroke volume	-	65 ml
Blood flow to Skin	-	10 ml/100gm
Weight of skin	-	2500 gm

1. What is the peculiar feature of blood flow to this organ?
2. What is the normal blood flow to this organ in one minute?

Answer

Cardiac output = SV × HR

= 72 × 65

= 4680 ml/min

Blood flow to skin = 100 gm – 10 ml

$= 2500 - \frac{250 \times 100}{4650}$

= 250 ml

% of cardiac output = 4650 – 100%

$= 250 - \frac{250 \times 100}{4650}$

= 5.3%

1. i. *Vasomotion:* Blood flow is of intermittent type due to itermittent contraction of meta-arterioles and pre capillary sphincter.
   ii. Arteriovenous anastomosis of cutaneous circulation enables thermoregulation to regulate the blood flow from 1 ml to 150 ml/100 gm/min.
   iii. *Blood reservoir:* Stores blood in the subdermal capillary and venous plexus.
2. 2.6 ml/100 gm/min.

CALCULATION 23

Calculate the percentage of cardiac output going to the muscle from the following data:

Heart rate	= 75/min
Stroke volume	= 70 ml
Blood flow to muscle	= 15 ml/100 gm
Weight of muscle	= 5000 gm

1. What is the peculiar feature of blood flow to this organ?
2. What is the normal blood flow to this organ in one minute?

Answer

Cardiac output = 75 × 70 = 5250 ml/min

Blood flow to muscle = 5000 × 15/100 = 750 ml/min

% of cardiac output = 750 × 100/5250 = 14%

1. a. Blood flow is phasic or intermittent in the contracting muscles being reduced during contraction due to compression of the arterioles and increased during muscle relaxation.
   b. Increase in blood flow during muscular exercise from 2–4 ml to 50–70 ml per 100 gm per min.
2. Normal blood flow to muscle is 2–4 ml/100 gm/min.

CALCULATION 24

Calculate the percentage of cardiac output going to the kidney from the following data:

Heart rate - 70/min

Stroke volume - 69 ml

Blood flow to Kidney - 900 ml/100 gm

Weight of kidney - 120 gm

1. What is the peculiar feature of blood flow to this organ?
2. What is the normal blood flow to this organ in one minute?

Answer

Cardiac output = HR × SV

= 70 × 69 = 4830 ml/min

Blood flow to kidney $= \frac{120 \times 900}{100}$

= 1080 ml/min.

% of cardiac out put = 4830 – 100%

$= 1080 - \frac{1080 \times 100}{100}$

= 22%

1. i. Renal arteries arise directly from abdominal aorta and hence it has higher renal hydrostatic capillary pressure of 60 mmHg.
   ii. Kidneys receive maximum blood flow about 1200 ml/min when compare to its weight.
   iii. Renal circulation has a portal system that is a double network of capillaries. Afferent arteriole → glomerular capillaries → efferent arteriole.

CALCULATION 25

Calculate the blood flow to the heart from the following data:

Heart rate - 70/min

Stroke volume - 70 ml

Percentage of cardiac output - 10%

1. What is the peculiar feature of blood flow to this organ?
2. What is the normal blood flow to this organ in one minute?

Answer

Cardiac output = Stroke volume × Heart rate

= 70 × 70 = 4900 ml.

Blood flow to heart $= \frac{8 \times 4900}{100} = 392$ ml/min.

1. i. They are end arteries.
   ii. It is the only organ in which maximum flow is received during diastole (phasic flow).
   iii. Heart is the only organ of the body that generates its own perfusion pressure (By autoregulation)
   iv. They have a high oxygen extraction ratio.
   2:200 to 250 ml/min.

CALCULATION 26

Calculate the blood flow to the kidney from the following data:

Heart rate - 70/min

Stroke volume - 68 ml

Percentage of cardiac output - 15.5%

1. What is the peculiar feature of blood flow to this organ?
2. What is the normal blood flow to this organ in one minute?

Answer

Cardiac output = Stroke volume × Heart rate

= 68 × 70 = 4760 ml.

Blood flow to Kidney $= \frac{15.5 \times 4760}{100}$

= 737 ml/min.

1. i. Renal arteries arise directly from abdominal aorta and hence they have higher renal hydrostatic pressure of 60 mmHg.
   ii. Kidneys are the second once to receive maximum blood flow about 1200 ml/min.
   iii. Renal circulation has a portal system that is a double network of capillaries. Afferent arteriole →

glomerular capillaries → efferent arteriole → peritubular capillaries.

iv. Autoregulation of blood flow is well established in kidneys in the range of 80 to 180 mmHg.

2. Normal blood flow to kidney is 1200 ml/min.

CALCULATION 27

Calculate the cardiac out put from the following data.

1. CO_2 given out/min = 240 ml
2. CO_2 content of mixed venous blood = 50 ml%
3. CO_2 content of arterial blood = 45 ml%

1. Define minute volume?
2. What is the normal value?
3. What method is used here?

Answer

$$\text{Cardiac out put} = \frac{CO_2 \text{ given out}}{\text{Arteriovenous } CO_2 \text{ difference}}$$

$$= \frac{240}{50 - 45} \times 100$$

$$= \frac{240}{5} \times 100$$

$$= 4800 \text{ ml/min.}$$

1. *Minute volume*

   Minute volume is the output of blood by the ventricle/mts.

2. Normal value = Stroke volume × Heart rate

   = 70 × 72 = 5.04 L/min

3. Fick's principle.

CALCULATION 28

Calculate the cardiac output from the following data:

1. O_2 uptake per minute = 250 ml
2. O_2 content of mixed venous blood = 20 ml%
3. O_2 content of arterial blood = 25 ml%

1. Define minute volume?
2. What is the normal value?
3. What method is used here?

Answer

$$\text{Cardiac output} = \frac{O_2 \text{ uptake / min}}{\text{Arteriovenous } O_2 \text{ difference}}$$

$$= \frac{250}{25 - 20} \times 100$$

$$= \frac{250}{5} \times 100 = 5000 \text{ ml/min}$$

1. *Minute volume:* Minute volume is the output of blood by the ventricle per minute.
2. Normal value = Stroke volume × Heart rate

   = 70 × 72 = 5.04 L/min

3. Fick's principle.

Reader's Notes

Reader's Notes

Reader's Notes